Facelift: Current Approaches

Guest Editor

STEPHEN PRENDIVILLE, MD

FACIAL PLASTIC SURGERY CLINICS OF NORTH AMERICA

www.facialplastic.theclinics.com

November 2009 • Volume 17 • Number 4

SAUNDERS an imprint of ELSEVIER, Inc.

W.B. SAUNDERS COMPANY
A Division of Elsevier Inc.

1600 John F. Kennedy Blvd., Suite 1800, Philadelphia, PA 19103-2899

http://www.theclinics.com

FACIAL PLASTIC SURGERY CLINICS OF NORTH AMERICA Volume 17, Number 4
November 2009 ISSN 1064-7406, ISBN 1-4377-1216-9, 978-1-4377-1216-2

Editor: Joanne Husovski
Developmental Editor: Donald Mumford

Facial Plastic Surgery Clinics of North America (ISSN 1064-7406) is published quarterly by Elsevier Inc., 360 Park Avenue South, New York, NY 10010-1710. Months of issue are February, May, August, and November. Business and Editorial Offices: 1600 John F. Kennedy Blvd., Suite 1800, Philadelphia, PA 19103-2899. Periodicals postage paid at New York, NY, and additional mailing offices. Subscription prices are $273.00 per year (US individuals), $428.00 per year (US institutions), $307.00 per year (Canadian individuals), $513.00 per year (Canadian institutions), $368.00 per year (foreign individuals), $513.00 per year (foreign institutions), $133.00 per year (US students), and $185.00 per year (foreign students). Foreign air speed delivery is included in all *Clinics* subscription prices. All prices are subject to change without notice. POSTMASTER: Send address changes to *Facial Plastic Surgery Clinics*, Elsevier Health Sciences Division, Subscription Customer Service, 3251 Riverport Lane, Maryland Heights, MO 63043. **Customer service: 1-800-654-2452 (US and Canada); 1-314-447-8871 (outside US and Canada); Fax: 314-447-8029; E-mail:journalscustomerservice-usa@elsevier.com (for print support); journalsonline support-usa@elsevier.com (for online support).**

Reprints. For copies of 100 or more of articles in this publication, please contact the Commercial Reprints Department, Elsevier Inc., 360 Park Avenue South, New York, NY 10010-1710. Tel.: 212-633-3812; Fax: 212-462-1935; E-mail: reprints@elsevier.com.

Facial Plastic Surgery Clinics of North America is covered in *MEDLINE*/PubMed (*Index Medicus*).

Printed and bound by CPI Group (UK) Ltd, Croydon, CR0 4YY
Transferred to Digital Print 2011

Contributors

GUEST EDITOR

STEPHEN PRENDIVILLE, MD
Southwest Florida Facial Plastic Surgery
Associates, Fort Myers, Florida

AUTHORS

SHAN R. BAKER, MD
Professor and Chief, Section of Facial Plastic
and Reconstructive Surgery, Department
of Otolaryngology-Head and Neck Surgery,
University of Michigan, Ann Arbor, Michigan;
Professor and Director, Center for Facial
Cosmetic Surgery, University of Michigan,
Livonia, Michigan

BENJAMIN A. BASSICHIS, MD, FACS
Medical Director, Advanced Facial Plastic
Surgery Center, Dallas, Texas

GARY BORODIC, MD
Surgeon, Massachusetts Eye and Ear Infirmary;
Assistant Clinical Professor, Harvard Medical
School, Boston, Massachusetts; Consultant,
Mentor Corporation, a Johnson and Johnson
Company, Santa Barbara, California

DAVID CAIRD, PhD
Ispen Pharma GmbH, Ettlingen, Germany

DAVID A. CAPLIN, MD
Clinical Instructor, Division of Parkcrest Plastic
Surgery, University of Washington, St Louis,
Missouri

ROSS A. CLEVENS, MD, FACS
Director of The Clevens Center for Facial
Cosmetic Surgery and Imperial Spa,
Melbourne, Merritt Island and Suntree,
Florida; Voluntary Faculty, University of
Central Florida College of Medicine,
Orlando, Florida

J. DAVID HOLCOMB, MD
Private Practice, Holcomb Facial Plastic
Surgery, Aesthetic Light and Laser Center,
Sarasota, Florida

AMIR M. KARAM, MD
Director, Carmel Valley Facial Plastic Surgery,
San Diego, California; Clinical faculty, Division
of Otolaryngology-Head and Neck Surgery,
Department of Surgery, University of California,
San Diego, California

SAMUEL M. LAM, MD
Director, Willow Bend Wellness Center & Lam
Facial Plastics, Plano, Texas

GRIGORIY MASHKEVICH, MD
Assistant Professor, Facial Plastic &
Reconstructive Surgery, Department of
Otolaryngology-Head & Neck Surgery, The
New York Eye & Ear Infirmary, New York,
New York

L. MIKE NAYAK, MD
Director, Nayak Plastic Surgery and Skin
Enhancement Center, St Louis, Missouri;
Clinical Assistant Professor, Department
of Otolaryngology-Head and Neck Surgery,
St Louis University, St Louis, Missouri

AMIT B. PATEL, MD
Assistant Professor of Surgery, University
of Kentucky-Albert Chandler Medical Center,
Meridian Plastic Surgeons, Indianapolis,
Indiana

STEPHEN W. PERKINS, MD
Meridian Plastic Surgeons, Indianapolis,
Indiana

CHAD A. PERLYN, MD, PhD
Florida International University, College
of Medicine, Miami, Florida

ANDY PICKETT, PhD
Biological Science and Technology, Ispen
Biopharm Limited, Wrexham, United Kingdom

STEPHEN PRENDIVILLE, MD
Southwest Florida Facial Plastic Surgery
Associates, Fort Myers, Florida

JEFFREY H. WACHHOLZ, MD
Chief of Otolaryngology (Facial Plastic
Surgery), Department of Otolaryngology,
St Vincent's Medical Center; President, The
Wachholz Clinic, P.A., 2700 Riverside
Avenue, Jacksonville, Florida

SETH WEISER, CRNA
Fort Myers, Sarasota, Florida

MARC S. ZIMBLER, MD
Director of Facial Plastic & Reconstructive
Surgery, Department of Otolaryngology-Head
& Neck Surgery, Beth Israel Medical Center,
Union Square East, New York, New York

Contents

Optimizing outcomes for rhytidectomy patients involves careful evaluation for conditions likely to benefit from adjunctive facial contouring and/or skin resurfacing procedures. On an individual basis, concurrent procedures should be performed only if benefits far outweigh any added risk and patient safety is not compromised. In this manner, physicians may improve practice productivity and overall patient satisfaction.

Facelift is the cornerstone procedure for the rejuvenation of the aging face. This procedure aims to improve the appearance of the lower two thirds of the face and neck. As with all surgical procedures, facelift is associated with certain risks and benefits. This article describes the sources of patient dissatisfaction and the avoidance and management of complications related to facelift surgery. A clinically oriented comprehensive review of the assessment and management of complications encountered during facelift surgery of the lower two thirds of the face and neck is presented.

Anesthesia for the patient undergoing facial plastic surgery can be approached in a variety of ways. This article describes a technique with which the authors have had great success. The principles of patient safety and comfort are essential elements in providing anesthesia for a facial plastic surgical case. A well-performed anesthetic makes a smooth postoperative course more likely, but a poorly handled anesthetic can increase the likelihood of postoperative complications and can strain the relationship between surgeon and patient. There cannot be enough emphasis on making and keeping the patient happy. A happy patient will do better in the long run, will be more willing to undergo future procedures, and often provides the best form of advertisement: word of mouth.

Cosmetic rejuvenation of the lower face can be accomplished effectively with facelift surgery; however, aesthetic outcomes are significantly improved when surgical traction combined with midface volume restoration is achieved and perpetuated. Incorporating the current understanding of the evolving process of facial maturation, this article puts forth an approach to full-face rejuvenation involving the continued treatment of the facelift patients with injectable filler materials for years after the surgical procedures. Beyond a three-dimensional approach, this "four-dimensional" method can achieve persistent, effective, natural-appearing outcomes that can be maintained successfully and dynamically over time.

loss, sun damage, and other causes. To achieve the patient's desired result, surgeons use various techniques, either in isolation or in combination. Careful preoperative evaluation of the patient's anatomy dictates the most appropriate procedure, ranging from laser skin resurfacing to sub-superficial muscular aponeurotic system (sub-SMAS) rhytidectomy with an extended platysmaplasty. This article reviews the techniques that are available and the decision-making process in choosing the appropriate technique for the individual patient.

The surgical management of the patient with the heavy face and neck requires an appreciation of the multiple anatomic and physiologic factors responsible for the associated displeasing appearance. Preoperative planning and patient selection are key components in achieving optimal outcomes. Furthermore, while approaches and techniques applied in traditional facelifts are beneficial, additional or modified maneuvers are often necessary to produce the desired outcomes in this challenging patient group.

This article addresses some of the nonsurgical considerations in caring for male patients. We are witnessing an ever-increasing level of interest in aesthetic surgery among men, and the unique considerations related to addressing male patients compared to female patients merit our attention. The care of male patients is characterized by important differences along each step of the surgical process. Men display a different set of motivations, concerns, and aesthetic ideals compared with women. Men also demonstrate decision-making processes and problem-solving approaches that contrast with approaches observed among women. These unique differences compel facial plastic surgeons to manage male patients differently from female patients.

Facelift surgery is complex and requires a significant commitment from both patient and surgeon. This article provides a collection of surgical tips and pearls that can be applied to most facelift procedures, no matter the surgical technique. A holistic approach to patient care is discussed regarding preoperative, perioperative, and postoperative management. Within this article the authors outline details so facial plastic surgeons can provide their patients with the smoothest surgical experience and recovery.

A discussion with Dr. Gary Borodic and Drs. Andy Pickett and David Caird on the long-term implications of cosmetic use of botox.

Facial Plastic Surgery Clinics of North America

THE CLINICS ARE NOW AVAILABLE ONLINE!

Access your subscription at:
www.theclinics.com

Preface

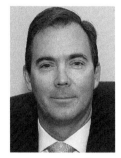

Stephen Prendiville, MD
Guest Editor

It is an honor and a privilege to serve as a Guest Editor for this edition of *Facial Plastic Surgery Clinics of North America*. The opportunity to share ideas with mentors and colleagues is thought provoking and exhilarating. Likewise, it represents an opportunity to stimulate intellectual and practical developments in surgical technique, patient management, and philosophy of practice.

Rhytidectomy or facelift techniques have been described in numerous ways over the last century, evolving from small incision, skin-based procedures, to SMAS-based techniques, deep-plane techniques, and subperiosteal techniques. In some ways, this wheel of surgical approaches is coming full circle with a return to less invasive procedures. Whether this represents evolution or devolution is currently an area of controversy. Ultimately, aesthetic outcomes, longevity of results, and overall patient satisfaction will be the deciders in this debate.

In the mind's eye of many facial plastic surgeons, rhytidectomy is a technique ostensibly designed to address aging changes in the midface, jawline, and neck. However, public understanding of the term "facelift" is seen more as an analogy for total facial rejuvenation. Increasingly, many surgeons are incorporating adjunctive techniques to help patients achieve their goals. In this way, facelift can be approached in a systematic approach (similar to our approach to rhinoplasty) toward the individual subcomponents that make up the procedure, using or omitting elements when and where indicated.

The purpose of this edition is to present a range of rationale-based approaches that can be used in facelift, recognizing that the proper technique must be applied for the right indications, and that certain tools in the armamentarium of facelift work more effectively in certain hands than others. Furthermore, this edition is intended to highlight elements of patient management that go beyond surgical technique and to enhance the surgical result with a pleasant patient experience.

I would like to thank all of the surgeons who have made contributions to this edition for their time and for sharing their expertise and thought process in applying various facelift techniques. Likewise, I would like to thank the readers of *Facial Plastic Surgery Clinics of North America* for a continued willingness to expand their intellectual horizons.

Stephen Prendiville, MD
9407, Cypress Lake Drive, Suite A
Fort Myers, FL 33919, USA

E-mail address:
StevePrendiville@msn.com

Facial Plast Surg Clin N Am 17 (2009) ix
doi:10.1016/j.fsc.2009.06.009

Facelift Adjunctive Techniques: Skin Resurfacing and Volumetric Contouring

J. David Holcomb, MD

KEYWORDS

- Facelift • Laser • Skin resurfacing
- Midface • Neck • Contouring

Posterior cervicofacial rhytidectomy is variably effective for reduction of jowling and improvement of mandibular contour, and may provide only limited temporary improvement of midface contour.[1,2] In predisposed patients, posterior cervicofacial rhytidectomy may worsen the appearance of midfacial (eg, submalar) volume loss.[3] Commonly employed posterior cervicofacial rhytidectomy (eg, superficial muscular aponeurotic system [SMAS]) approaches may minimally efface[4] or may even accentuate melolabial fold depth.[5] Posterior cervicofacial rhytidectomy may also result in discordant facial rejuvenation if intrinsic skin aging and age-related changes of the forehead, periorbital and perioral areas, and submentum and neck are not also addressed. In addition, improvements in mandibular and midface contour obtained via rhytidectomy generally diminish over time as tissues undergo stress relaxation and gravitational changes postoperatively[1]– changes that are typically greater in patients with more advanced chronologic age, advanced skin photoaging or heavier body habitus, and in those with a history of smoking or significant weight loss. Optimization of facial rejuvenation outcomes therefore requires meticulous execution of rhytidectomy techniques while also addressing skin photoaging, rhytidosis, and idiosyncratic age-related volumetric tissue changes.

ADJUNCTIVE PROCEDURES OF MIDDLE FACIAL THIRD

Posterior cervicofacial SMAS imbrication or plication rhytidectomy procedures may not adequately address age-related structural changes in the midface including malar fat pad descent, melolabial fold ptosis, and submalar volume loss. Alternative rhytidectomy procedures conceived to enhance midface outcomes (eg, improve effacement of melolabial fold with composite facelift,[4] deep plane facelift,[6] extended SMAS facelift with direct plication of the malar fat pad,[7] subperiosteal midface lift[8]) have not met universal acceptance as a result of variable efficacy and increased surgical risk. Certain adjunctive procedures are commonly performed with posterior cervicofacial rhytidectomy. Concurrent subperiosteal submalar augmentation effectively reverses submalar insufficiency and provides long-term improvement of midface contour.[9] Concurrent midface soft tissue augmentation (eg, via filler injections, autologous fat transfer, or SMAS graft[10]) may provide temporary improvement of relative midface volume loss (created in part by osseous midface changes[11–13] and malar fat pad descent[2,4,7,8,10]) and partially camouflage descended fat at the melolabial fold. Even though increasing benefit (greater camouflage of anatomic correlates of descended fat) may be obtained with secondary and tertiary

By way of disclosure some of the following may be pertinent regarding my relationship with Lutronic Inc: Medical Advisory Board, Equipment Discount, Honoraria, Stock Options.

Holcomb Facial Plastic Surgery, Aesthetic Light and Laser Center, 1 S. School Avenue, Ste 800, Sarasota, FL 34237, USA

E-mail address: drholcomb@srqfps.com

Facial Plast Surg Clin N Am 17 (2009) 505–514
doi:10.1016/j.fsc.2009.06.012
1064-7406/09/$ – see front matter © 2009 Elsevier Inc. All rights reserved.

autologous fat grafting procedures, the primary underlying problem (descended fat) remains unaddressed.

Mobilization of ptotic malar fat pad tissues during subperiosteal midface lifting may not sufficiently efface the melolabial folds or recruit or adequately fixate enough tissue to provide long-term improvement of midface contour.[2,8,10] As early as 1989 McKinney and Cook advocated lipocontouring of the nasolabial fold during facelift surgery.[14] Despite reporting consistent synergistic improvement in the midface, the technique did not become popularized.

Nonetheless, the idea that substantial aesthetic improvement of the midface may be obtained via tissue removal as opposed to tissue repositioning or soft tissue augmentation is an intriguing concept. Although still early in its inception, an appealing alternative to repositioning displaced midface fat or to camouflage of the anatomic correlates of displaced midface fat involves use of a novel 1444-nm Nd-YAG lipolysis laser (see later discussion).

Preoperative evaluation of the aging midface should address the suborbital, malar, submalar, melolabial fold, or lip cheek groove, and the maxillary dentoalveolar structures. Aesthetic rejuvenation of the midface must at a minimum attempt to restore volume in the suborbital, malar, and submalar areas, and to improve the contour of the medial cheek. Transblepharoplasty or transoral alloplastic augmentation or transcutaneous or transoral injection with hyaluronic acid or calcium hydroxylapetite filler materials should be considered for suborbital insufficiency. Transoral alloplastic augmentation should be considered for malar, submalar, and combined malar-submalar insufficiency. Although modest correction of malar and/or submalar insufficiency may be obtained with injectable filler materials, results with alloplastic implants are generally superior both in volumetric correction and longevity of results. Patients with loss of maxillary alveolar height and volume may exhibit greater caudal midfacial volume loss for which optimum correction may require alloplastic implants, soft tissue augmentation, and dentoalveolar correction (eg, prosthetic denture).

SUBMALAR AUGMENTATION

Transoral placement of submalar implants should immediately follow rhytidectomy to minimize any risk of cross contamination and wound infection. Transoral submalar implant placement requires significantly less dissection for pocket creation than for placement of a malar or combined malar-submalar implant. The dissection should extend anterior to the masseter muscle fibers and superolaterally over the distal zygoma to create a pocket just large enough to accept the implant. On completion of undermining, use of sterile implant sizers allows determination of final implant shape and size. The pocket should be irrigated with antibiotic-containing solution before placement of the implant. Fixation is not generally required for submalar implant placement. The procedure has high patient satisfaction, is relatively quick and has a low complication rate.

LASER LIPOLYSIS-ASSISTED FACIAL CONTOURING: MELOLABIAL FOLD

Retrusion of the anterior maxilla and enlargement of the pyriform aperture contribute to midfacial soft tissue sagging and deepening of the melolabial fold.[12-14] Remote procedures designed to reposition ptotic midfacial soft tissues have been variably effective at best.[8] Empirically, it follows that direct reduction of ptotic midfacial soft tissue should be highly effective.[2] Although not commonly performed because of the need for a lengthy incision, direct excision of the melolabial fold (debulking of ptotic skin and fat) is unparalleled for effective rejuvenation of the medial cheek. An emerging alternative involves laser-assisted volumetric contouring of the melolabial fold with a novel 1444-nm Nd-YAG fiber laser.

Compared with other wavelengths currently used for laser lipolysis (eg, 1064 nm, 1320 nm) the 1444-nm Nd-YAG laser offers numerous advantages that arise from greater specificity for subcutaneous fat and tissue water.[15] **Fig. 1** shows the absorption curves for fat and water for the most common lipolysis laser wavelengths. The greater selectivity of the 1444-nm lipolysis laser provides improved efficiency and greater thermal confinement[15] (energy relatively more localized near source, ie, tip of laser fiber), which are extremely important features that enable safe use of this technology for subregional facial contouring. With reduced thermal diffusivity (a relative measure of thermal conduction through tissue, in this case, fat) and decreased energy requirement for lipolysis, the 1444-nm lipolysis laser may be used in areas where tissues are delicate and where there exists a corresponding need to limit nonspecific collateral tissue damage.

Subregional facial volumetric tissue contouring assisted by 1444-nm lipolysis laser may be performed concurrent with or independent of rhytidectomy procedures. Treatment areas include the medial cheek (melolabial fold area), caudal

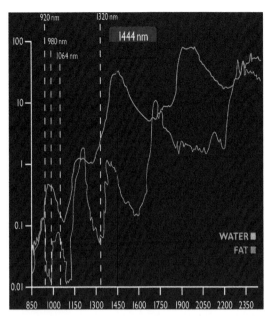

Fig. 1. Fat and water optical absorption curves for various laser wavelengths (x-axis, wavelength in nanometers; y-axis, optical absorption on logarithmic scale). Vertical lines identify wavelengths currently in use for laser lipolysis.

cheek at jawline (jowl area), and submentum and neck.

Lipolysis laser-assisted facial contouring involves 5 basic steps:

1. Creation of a small access wound for entry of the laser fiber
2. Infiltration of local anesthetic or tumescent solution
3. Delivery of laser energy to the target tissue
4. Aspiration of partially emulsified and liquefied fat
5. Closure of the access wound

Before lasing, the device is programmed with power (watts), pulse energy (mJ), pulse frequency (Hz), and total energy (J) for the designated treatment area. After the fiber is introduced, the surgeon begins lasing. Laser energy delivery stops at the discretion of the surgeon or continues until the total preset energy is expended (the device counts down toward zero). Aspiration of partially emulsified and liquefied fat is then performed with a small cannula attached to a 5-mL syringe prefilled with 1 mL of sterile saline. For paired or bilateral treatment areas, the procedure is repeated on the contralateral side in identical fashion using the same total energy and other laser settings, and with aspiration of a similar volume of fat (unless there is significant preexisting asymmetry).

Fig. 2A–D (this patient did not undergo concurrent rhytidectomy) shows the intra-operative steps

outlined earlier for 1444-nm Nd-YAG laser-assisted subregional facial volumetric tissue contouring at the melolabial fold. The steps are identical whether completed independent of or concurrent with rhytidectomy techniques. **Fig. 3A–D** shows before and after photographs for revision posterior cervicofacial SMAS imbrication rhytidectomy, trichophytic browlift and transcutaneous lower blepharoplasty with concurrent 1444-nm Nd-YAG laser-assisted subregional facial volumetric tissue contouring (at the melolabial fold), and laser-assisted submentoplasty and perioral erbium-YAG laser skin resurfacing.

The 1444-nm Nd-YAG laser may also be used to pre-dissect the cervicofacial rhytidectomy flap wherein the fiber is passed back and forth and in a criss-cross fashion to evenly heat the immediate subdermal tissues and thereby lyse some of the attachments between the hypodermis and upper subcutis. **Fig. 4A–D** illustrates this process; **Fig. 4E, F** are preoperative and postoperative photographs for posterior cervicofacial SMAS imbrication rhytidectomy with concurrent 1444-nm Nd-YAG laser-assisted subregional facial volumetric tissue contouring (at the melolabial fold), and perioral ablative fractional CO_2 laser resurfacing. This technique does seem to reduce the time and physical effort necessary to elevate the cervicofacial rhytidectomy flap. A randomized multicenter study is currently underway to evaluate its merits.

Candidates for laser lipolysis-assisted contouring of the melolabial fold include patients with mild, moderate, or severe ptosis of the melolabial fold and may include (1) patients considering concurrent rhytidectomy, (2) patients considering filler injections, (3) patients who are poor candidates for rhytidectomy procedures or filler injections. If performed concurrent with facelift, laser lipolysis-assisted contouring of the melolabial fold should be performed immediately preceding posterior cervicofacial rhytidectomy to allow for any additional movement of the skin envelope afforded by the contouring procedure.

Benefits observed from laser lipolysis-assisted contouring of the melolabial fold include decreased melolabial fold depth and ptosis, improved malar emanence highlight, improved lower eyelid-cheek junction transition and submalar triangle aesthetics, and reduced appearance of midfacial relative volume loss. This adjunctive technique may reduce or modify the need for midface and perioral soft tissue augmentation, and provide some further tightening of the midfacial skin soft tissue envelope. The removal of descended fat is permanent but the long-term results and benefits of this technique remain to be

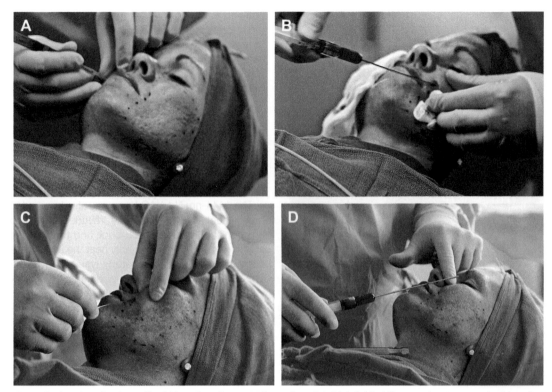

Fig. 2. Basic steps for laser lipolysis-assisted contouring of melolabial fold: (*A*) very short access incision (eg, 1.5 mm); (*B*) infiltration of local anesthetic (eg, 0.5% lidocaine, 0.25% marcaine, 1:200,000 epinephrine, Hyaluronidase (Vitrase) 4 IU/mL) using multihole infiltrator (eg, Tulip 1.6 mm); (*C*) laser lipolysis with 1444-nm Nd-YAG laser (600-mm bare fiber); (*D*) limited mechanical aspiration with multihole cannula (eg, Tulip 2.1 mm Tri-Port) and 5 mL syringe prefilled with 1 mL of normal saline.

determined. Nonetheless, laser lipolysis-assisted contouring of the melolabial fold seems to be an extremely promising adjunctive technique for midface rejuvenation.

Anticipated treatment sequelae observed to date include ecchymosis, edema, hypoesthesia of the skin overlying the treatment area, tenderness of the treatment area during initial healing. Unanticipated treatment complications (eg, infection at treatment site, insufficient skin tightening, hematoma, overcorrection with contour irregularity, minor thermal injury at entry site, non–entry site full-thickness cutaneous burn and seroma) should be rare if appropriate techniques are followed. Nonetheless, several minor complications have been observed in 2 initial study centers (Sarasota, Florida and Seoul, Korea). Minor thermal injury (second-degree burn) of the skin immediately adjacent to the fiber entry site has been observed on several occasions. The affected areas healed uneventfully with appropriate wound care. Infection was also observed at a single surgical site that was determined to be secondary to interiorization of a cutaneous cyst. The skin over laser lipolysis-assisted contouring treatment areas

should be carefully evaluated preoperatively and any significant cystic lesions should be removed before any skin undermining with a fiber laser.

ADJUNCTIVE PROCEDURES OF LOWER FACIAL THIRD

Although posterior cervicofacial rhytidectomy is generally very effective for reduction of jowling, results generally diminish over time as tissues undergo stress relaxation and gravitational changes postoperatively;[1] these changes are typically greater in patients with more advanced chronologic age, advanced skin photoaging, or heavier body habitus, and in patients with a history of smoking or significant weight loss. In the lower third of the face, features of aging, changes in mandibular osseous volume and contour over the parasymphyseal regions and anterior mentum tend to acutely worsen the appearance of jowling, marionette lines, and submental soft tissue excess and ptosis.[16–18] Aging of the lips with loss of volume and decreased vermillion show also profoundly affect facial appearance.[19] If pronounced, failure to address these changes in

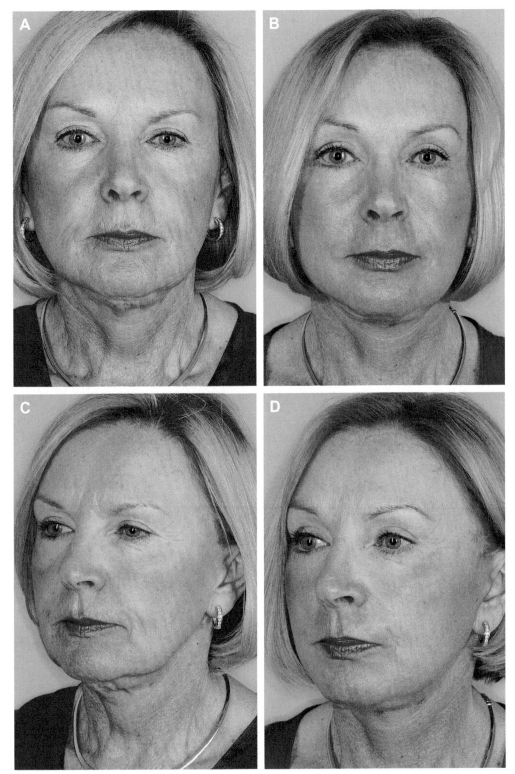

Fig. 3. Frontal (*A*, *B*) and oblique (*C*, *D*) before (*A*, *C*) and after (*B*, *D*) photographs following trichophytic browlift, lower blepharoplasty, posterior cervicofacial SMAS imbrication rhytidectomy, 1444-nm Nd-YAG laser-assisted contouring of melolabial fold, perioral erbium-YAG laser (single pass ablate + coagulate, Sciton tunable resurfacing laser) skin resurfacing. The 1444-nm Nd-YAG laser was also used to pre-dissect (partially undermine) posterior cervicofacial rhytidectomy flaps.

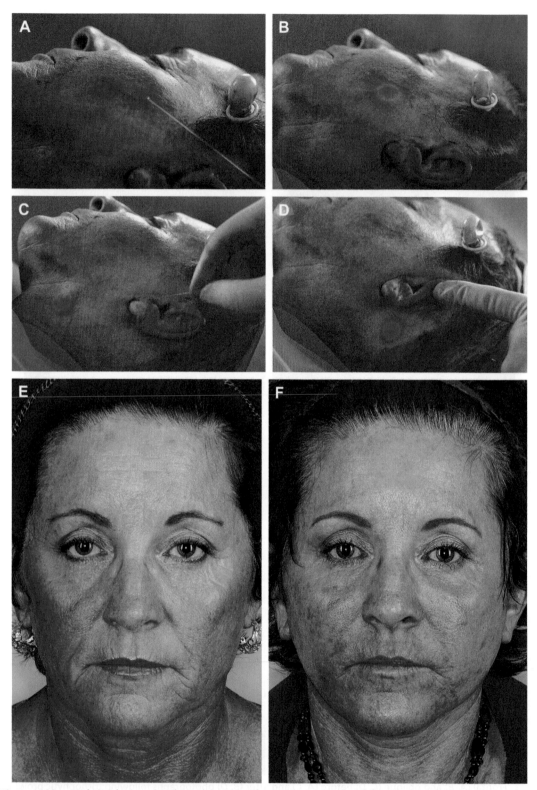

Fig. 4. 1444-nm Nd-YAG laser-assisted pre-dissection of posterior cervicofacial rhytidectomy flap. (*A*) 600-mm bare laser fiber over cheek; (*B, C, D*) laser fiber pre-dissection of cheek, neck, and postauricular areas); (*E*) preoperative and (*F*) postoperative frontal photographs following posterior cervicofacial SMAS imbrication rhytidectomy and perioral fractional CO_2 laser (300-mm and 120-mm spot sizes, Lutronic eCO_2) skin resurfacing.

the lips may have a negative effect on facial rejuvenation outcomes.

Preoperative evaluation of the aging lower third of the face should address lip volume, vermillion show, angulation of the oral commissure, nasolabial angle, columella and nasal tip rotation, and soft tissue ptosis and volumetric changes of the bony mentum and parasymphyseal regions.

Loss of lip volume may be improved with filler injections, autologous tissue transfer (eg, SMAS) or alloplastic implants.[19] Although lip augmentation typically improves vermillion show, advancement of the vermillion is an extremely effective option that avoids the need for repeated filler injections and the potential long-term problems occasionally encountered with alloplastic implants.[20] Acute downward angulation of the oral commissure may be improved with procedures that elevate the corner of the mouth and may be incorporated with upper lip vermillion advancement.

Gradual loss of nasal tip support tends to decrease nasal tip rotation and nasolabial angle. If pronounced, correction of tip ptosis or hanging columella significantly improves the aesthetics of the upper lip region.

Osseous pre-jowl insufficiency tends to worsen the appearance of jowling and somewhat diminish the impact of posterior cervicofacial rhytidectomy procedures if not addressed.[18] Options for correction include calcium hydroxylapetite or other filler injections and alloplastic implants for isolated pre-jowl insufficiency or combined insufficiency of the anterior mentum and pre-jowl areas.

ALLOPLASTIC AUGMENTATION

Correction of microgenia with or without associated pre-jowl insufficiency may be completed transorally or via an external approach.[16–18] Because most patients requesting chin augmentation also request contouring of the submentum and neck, an external approach via submental crease incision is more commonly performed. An external approach also minimizes the potential for wound contamination with intraoral pathogens. Care should be taken to avoid creation of a very large pocket if a non-fixated implant is used. Subperiosteal dissection should carefully continue laterally along the caudal margin of the lateral mentum and anterior mandibular body to avoid injury to the mandibular branch of the trigeminal nerve as it exits the mental foramen. On completion of subperiosteal undermining, use of sterile implant sizers allows determination of implant shape and size. The pocket should be irrigated with antibiotic solution before placement of the implant. Depending on implant type and anatomic fit, fixation with a titanium lag screw or initial suture fixation with stabilization to deep soft tissues may be necessary.

LASER LIPOLYSIS-ASSISTED FACIAL CONTOURING: JAWLINE (JOWL)

In predisposed patients (eg, heavier features, loss of tissue elasticity) jowling may not be sufficiently corrected or may partially return relatively soon after surgery.[1] Even if the skin flap has been extended and elevated over this area, the fibroadipose nature of the jowl is somewhat resistant to contouring with gentle liposuction (eg, single port cannula). Although occasionally discussed, open contouring and direct excision of the jowl is not a common practice.

An emerging alternative involves use of a novel 1444-nm Nd-YAG fiber laser for volumetric contouring of the jowl. The characteristics of the 1444-nm lipolysis laser enabling safe subregional facial volumetric tissue contouring have been discussed in an earlier section of this article. If performed during posterior cervicofacial rhytidectomy, contouring of the jowl with the 1444-nm Nd-YAG lipolysis laser does not require creation of a separate access wound for introduction of the laser fiber. Again, the device is programmed with power (watts), energy (mJ) and total energy (J) for the ipsilateral treatment area before lasing. After starting, lasing continues until the total preset energy is expended (the device counts down from preset total energy). After aspiration of partially emulsified and liquefied fat, the procedure is repeated in identical fashion on the contralateral side using the same total energy and other laser settings, and with aspiration of a similar volume of fat on both sides.

As an envisioned complementary procedure during posterior cervicofacial rhytidectomy, subregional contouring of the lower cheek and jowl area should be performed before mobilization and imbrication or plication of the SMAS to allow for any additional movement of the skin envelope afforded by the contouring procedure. Candidates for the procedure include patients undergoing rhytidectomy who also have significant subcutaneous fullness of the jowls (as opposed to predominant skin laxity). Subregional contouring of the lower cheek and jowl may also be performed as an isolated procedure separate from rhytidectomy as an alternative or complementary procedure to caudal melomental fold (pre-jowl sulcus) filler injections.

ADJUNCTIVE SKIN REJUVENATION

Wrinkles rank near the top of the list of leading concerns among patients seeking facial rejuvenation. Many studies have previously addressed the merits of skin rejuvenation and surgical facial rejuvenation with combinations including concurrent treatment with chemical exfoliants (phenol peel variations,[21] tricholoacetic acid[22]), lasers[23] (CO_2, erbium-YAG) and nitrogen plasma.[23] With the recent proliferation of laser devices, changing patient demographics (both younger and older, and patients of greater ethnic diversity seeking rejuvenation), and advancing concepts in skin rejuvenation, more studies evaluating concurrent therapies will certainly be forthcoming.

Concurrent rejuvenation of skin at remote, non-undermined facial areas (eg, perioral resurfacing with posterior cervicofacial rhytidectomy) does not pose any particular increased risk at the surgical site (rhytidectomy flap in this example).[23] Controversy exists regarding the safety of concurrent skin rejuvenation over surgical sites, especially for procedures involving significant tissue undermining and mobilization (see later discussion).

Patients' perception of outcomes (in number of years younger in appearance) shifts more significantly when skin rejuvenation is performed with (concurrent versus staged) surgical facial rejuvenation.[24] Other advantages of concurrent skin rejuvenation and surgical facial rejuvenation include avoidance of additional expense (eg, anesthesia and facility fees for staged resurfacing procedure) and down time.[23] Potential disadvantages of concurrent skin rejuvenation include compromised healing, worsened appearance in immediate postoperative period and greater complexity of wound care.[23]

Empirically, the safety margin for concurrent skin rejuvenation would seem to be:

1. Greatest over areas or regions remote from surgical sites
2. Very high for procedures that involve deep undermining (eg, subperiosteal undermining for placement of facial implants or endoscopic procedures)
3. Intermediate for procedures that involve less skin undermining and thicker flaps (eg, deep plane rhytidectomy approach)
4. Least for procedures that involve extensive skin undermining and mobilization of thinner flaps (eg, "mini" posterior cheek lift)

However, various factors such as extent of undermining of skin flap, thickness of skin flap, skin flap closure tension, history of smoking, type of skin resurfacing treatment, and numerous procedure-specific skin resurfacing variables potentially affect safety, and must also be weighed in consideration of concurrent skin rejuvenation and surgical facial rejuvenation.[23]

Clearly, deep phenol peels should not be performed concurrently over undermined flaps. Medium chemical peels, however, may be safely performed over undermined skin with primary short-term benefits of improved skin tone and superficial texture. Laser skin rejuvenation and, more recently, nitrogen plasma skin regeneration, have been the subject of intense interest as a concurrent modality for improving outcomes among facial rejuvenation patients.

Many factors affect laser skin tissue interaction. This discussion does not include nonablative laser skin rejuvenation because multiple treatments are necessary and typical benefits from a single treatment are far less than would be expected from a single concurrent ablative laser or nitrogen plasma treatment. Because resurfacing (ablative laser or nitrogen plasma) is well tolerated over areas remote from surgical sites or over areas of deep undermining, the remainder of this discussion focuses on the safety of such treatments over undermined tissue (eg, posterior cervicofacial rhytidectomy flap [PCFRF]).

CO_2 laser skin rejuvenation has been extensively evaluated for safety and effectiveness concurrent with aesthetic facial surgery including treatment of the undermined PCFRF.[23] Although some variation in technique exists among studies, such as extent of skin flap undermining and approach (eg, SMAS imbrication, composite or deep plane approach) and laser treatment parameters (eg, power, pulse energy, spot size, scan pattern, number of passes), concurrent CO_2 laser resurfacing of the undermined PCFRF has been generally safe with favorable outcomes.[23] Nonetheless, as popularity of full face, ablative, traditional (nonfractionated) CO_2 laser resurfacing has diminished, many practitioners have either limited (eg, single pass with lower fluences) or abandoned CO_2 laser resurfacing of the undermined PCFRF. Other practitioners have continued to perform concurrent skin resurfacing, including the undermined PCFRF, with other technologies including erbium-YAG lasers and nitrogen plasma skin regeneration. Proponents of erbium-YAG laser treatment suggest that tissue rearrangement associated with posterior cervicofacial rhytidectomy effectively smoothes deeper rhytids obviating the need for aggressive treatment of the undermined PCFRF.[25] In addition, such treatment effectively treats superficial dyschromias and photodamage and improves skin surface texture.

Although advantageous because of the shorter recovery period (compared with even single pass CO_2 laser treatment), benefits related to neocollagenesis are more limited with the extremely narrow zone of residual thermal damage (RTD) that results from short pulse erbium-YAG laser skin resurfacing.[25] Second-generation erbium-YAG lasers with long or variable extended pulse widths enable CO_2 laser-like effects with a substantial increase in RTD, but few practitioners advocate aggressive treatment of the undermined PCFRF. Depth of RTD, however, may be more carefully controlled with third-generation erbium-YAG laser resurfacing technology, which enables more precise user-controlled blending of pulse widths. Of particular advantage in the treatment of the undermined PCFRF, this feature may be used to achieve (superficial) ablation (of the epidermis) and (deeper) coagulation extending into the superficial dermis to enhance the overall effect with respect to collagen remodeling and skin tightening. The end result of this approach may be similar to the effects that can be achieved with aggressive treatment using a slightly different wavelength (2790-nm erbium-YSGG).

Proponents of nitrogen plasma skin regeneration contend that the unique features of this technology enable safe treatment of the undermined PCFRF with an even more favorable healing profile and enhanced depth of effect (versus single-pass ablative laser resurfacing).[23] Detailed evaluation of nitrogen plasma skin regeneration has demonstrated safe combination (concurrent) with aesthetic facial surgery for various procedures in the forehead, periorbital, midface, and perioral areas.[23] Despite full thickness coagulative injury that extends into the upper dermis, initial preservation of the epidermis and the absence of an open wound during neocollagenesis may minimize any added risk of infection during the early postoperative period while also lessening the complexity of skin care.[23]

Whereas nonablative fractional laser skin resurfacing seems largely nonmeritorious as a single concurrent therapy during aesthetic facial surgery, ablative fractional laser skin resurfacing should be explored as a concurrent therapy. Many factors affect ablative fractional laser skin tissue interaction including:

○ Wavelength
○ Spot size (incident at tissue)
○ Percent skin coverage (related to spot density or dot pitch)
○ Treatment depth
○ Pulse energy
○ Pulse width

○ Static versus dynamic treatment mode
○ Single versus multipulse energy delivery
○ Number of passes

Many of these treatment parameters are also inter-related, for example, with treatment depth affected by spot size and pulse energy and extended pulse width affecting percent skin coverage as a result of its effects on both micro-ablative column width and peripheral RTD.

Generally, if one is cautious regarding depth of treatment and percent skin coverage, concurrent treatment of the undermined PCFRF with any of the CO_2, erbium-YAG, or erbium-YSGG ablative fractional lasers is likely safe. Among other things, and similar to nitrogen plasma skin regeneration, ablative fractional laser resurfacing (all wavelengths) enables treatment of an extended range of Fitzpatrick skin types.[26,27] Formal studies evaluating the merits of and appropriate settings for such concurrent therapy would be a valuable addition to the literature.

Achieving optimum skin rejuvenation results with minimum risk may at times require blending of skin resurfacing modalities. Ablative CO_2 and erbium-YAG lasers have been used in combination previously (not as a concurrent therapy) with initial passes with either the CO_2 or erbium-YAG laser and the final pass with the erbium-YAG or CO_2 laser.[28,29] In this way RTD may be minimized such that laser skin resurfacing results are not compromised while also enabling more rapid healing. This concept may be extended to ablative fractional resurfacing (AFR) and erbium-YAG laser resurfacing wherein deep dermal ablation effected with single-pass CO_2 AFR is immediately followed by single or dual pulse mode (multiplexed short and long pulse) single-pass erbium-YAG laser resurfacing. For nonundermined skin this combination combines the tightening effect of CO_2 AFR with single-pass erbium-YAG resurfacing for partial to complete ablation of the epidermis and optional additional thermal injury to the upper dermis to further improve neocollagenesis and dermal remodeling. This blended laser skin resurfacing treatment modality seems to provide very adequate skin tightening and rhytid reduction, and maximum improvement of brown dyschromias and surface texture while also maintaining a favorable healing profile and minimum risk of complications. It will be interesting to see whether pure CO_2 AFR using a blend of spot sizes (eg, 300 mm and 120 mm) may also achieve these results.

SUMMARY

In summary, optimizing outcomes for rhytidectomy patients involves careful evaluation for conditions likely to benefit from adjunctive facial contouring and/or skin resurfacing procedures. On an individual basis, concurrent procedures should be performed only if benefits far outweigh any added risk and patient safety is not compromised. In this manner, physicians may improve practice productivity and overall patient satisfaction.

REFERENCES

1. Kamer FM. Sequential rhytidectomy and the two stage concept. Otolaryngol Clin North Am 1980; 13(2):305–20.

2. Hamra ST. A study of the long-term effect of malar fat repositioning in face lift surgery: short-term success but long-term failure. Plast Reconstr Surg 2002; 110(3):940–51.

3. Binder WJ, Schoenrock LD. Augmenation of the malar-submalar/midface. Facial Plast Surg Clin North Am 1994;2(3):265–83.

4. Hamra ST. Composite rhytidectomy. Plast Reconstr Surg 1992;90(1):1–13.

5. Barton FE. The SMAS and the nasolabial fold. Plast Reconstr Surg 1992;89(6):1054–7.

6. Alsarraf R, To WC, Johnson CM Jr, et al. The deep plane facelift. Facial Plast Surg 2003;19(1):95–106.

7. Owsley JQ. Face lift. Plast Reconstr Surg 1997; 100(2):514–9.

8. Williams EF III, Vargas H, Dahiya R, et al. Midfacial rejuvenation via a minimal-incision brow-lift approach: critical evaluation of a 5-year experience. Arch Facial Plast Surg 2003;5(6):470–8.

9. Binder WJ. A comprehensive approach for aesthetic contouring of the midface in rhytidectomy. Facial Plast Surg Clin North Am 1993;1(2):231–55.

10. Calderon W, Andrades PR, Israel GI, et al. SMAS graft of the nasolabial area during deep plane rhytidectomy. Plast Reconstr Surg 2004;114(2):559–64.

11. Pessa JE, Zadoo VP, Mutimer KL, et al. Relative maxillary retrusion as a natural consequence of aging: combining skeletal and soft-tissue changes into an integrated model of midfacial aging. Plast Reconstr Surg 1998;102(1):205–12.

12. Shaw RB, Kahn DM. Aging of the midface bony elements: a three dimensional CT study. Plast Reconstr Surg 2007;119(2):675–81.

13. Medelson BC, Jacobson SR. Age-related changes of the orbit and midcheek and the implications for facial rejuvenation. Aesthetic Plast Surg 2007; 31(5):419–23.

14. McKinney P, Cook JQ. Liposuction and the treatment of nasolabial folds. Aesthetic Plast Surg 1989;13(3): 167–71.

15. Youn J-I. A wavelength dependence study of laser-assisted lipolysis effect [abstract]. American Society for Laser Medicine and Surgery, 2009.

16. Romo T III, Yalamanchili H, Scalfani AP, et al. Chin and pre-jowl augmentation in the management of the aging jawline. Facial Plast Surg 2005;21(1): 38–46.

17. Mittelman H, Spencer JR, Chrzanowski DS, et al. Chin region: management of grooves and mandibular hypoplasia with alloplastic implants. Facial Plast Surg Clin North Am 2007;15(4):445–60.

18. Shire JR. The importance of the prejowl notch in face lifting: the prejowl implant. Facial Plast Surg Clin North Am 2008;16(1):87–97.

19. Segall L, Ellis D. Therapeutic options for lip augmentation. Facial Plast Surg Clin North Am 2007;15(4): 485–90.

20. Perkins NW, Smith SP Jr, Williams EF III, et al. Perioral rejuvenation: complementary techniques and procedures. Facial Plast Surg Clin North Am 2007; 15(4):423–32.

21. Dingman DL, Hartog J, Siemionow M, et al. Simultaneous deep plane facelift and trichloroacetic acid peel. Plast Reconstr Surg 1994;93(1):86–93.

22. Becker FF. Circumoral chemical peel combined with cervicofacial rhytidectomy. Arch Otolaryngol 1983; 109(3):172–4.

23. Holcomb JD, Kent KJ, Rousso DE, et al. Nitrogen plasma skin regeneration and aesthetic facial surgery: multicenter evaluation of concurrent treatment. Arch Facial Plast Surg 2009;11(3):1–10.

24. Roberts TL III, Pozner JN, Ritter E, et al. The RSVP facelift: a highly vascular flap permitting safe, simultaneous, comprehensive facial rejuvenation in one operative setting. Aesthetic Plast Surg 2000;24(5): 313–22.

25. Weinstein C, Pozner J, Schelflan M, et al. Combined erbium:YAG laser resurfacing and face lifting. Plast Reconstr Surg 2001;107(2):586–92.

26. Jih MH, Kimyai-Asadi A. Fractional photothermolysis: a review and update. Semin Cutan Med Surg 2008;27(1):63–71.

27. Alexiades-Armenakas MR, Dover JS, Arndt KA, et al. The spectrum of laser skin resurfacing: nonablative, fractional and ablative laser resurfacing. J Am Acad Dermatol 2008;58(5):719–37.

28. Millman AL, Mannor GE. Histologic and clinical evaluation of combined eyelid erbium:YAG and CO2 laser resurfacing. Am J Ophthalmol 1999;127(5): 614–6.

29. Fitzpatrick RE. Maximizing benefits and minimizing risk with CO2 laser resurfacing. Dermatol Clin 2002;20(1):77–86.

Avoiding Patient Dissatisfaction and Complications in Facelift Surgery

Ross A. Clevens, MD, FACS[a,b],*

KEYWORDS

- Facelift • Necklift • Complications • Unfavorable result
- Hematoma • Infection • Scarring • Alopecia

Facelift is the cornerstone procedure within the armamentarium of the aesthetic facial surgeon. This procedure rejuvenates the lower two thirds of the face and neck achieving a more youthful jawline and neckline. As with all surgical procedures, facelift or rhytidectomy is associated with certain risks and benefits including bleeding, infection, scarring, nerve injury, and failure to achieve a satisfactory outcome. This article describes the sources of patient dissatisfaction, and the avoidance, recognition, and management of certain common complications related to facelift surgery. Attention is focused on avoiding and managing complications during the preoperative, intraoperative, and postoperative care of the facelift patient. This article strives to be practical and technique related and aims to help the practicing facial plastic surgeon achieve excellence in facelift surgery. To facilitate the clinical applicability of this article, it is divided into considerations related to the preoperative, intraoperative, and postoperative care of the facelift patient.

PREOPERATIVE CONCERNS IN FACELIFT
Psychologic Considerations

There are numerous considerations in the evaluation of the facelift patient. Aesthetic surgery is unique as compared with other surgical disciplines because psychologic considerations weigh heavily in the approach to the surgical candidate. Unlike other branches of medicine and surgery, the facelift patient presents as an elective surgical candidate who has self-selected for surgical consideration. The facial plastic surgeon must assess the goals and expectations of the prospective facelift patient. A surgeon's first impressions of a patient often prove valuable for gauging the suitability of a surgical procedure. This assessment should take into consideration the motivators, recent life events, and reasonableness of the patient's anticipated outcome with regard to the planned surgery.

There are numerous formal and informal methods of assessing the patient's mental well-being. Formal evaluation includes standardized testing, such as the Minnesota Multiphasic Personality Inventory, California Personality Inventory, and Eysenck Personality Inventory. Numerous studies have found that such inventories yield inconsistent results and fail to detect psychopathologic patients. Additionally, such testing is impractical and cumbersome in a clinical practice.

Experienced clinicians suggest that the most effective method of assessing a patient's psychologic suitability is to spend time with the patient gathering information and forming an impression. Additionally, the candid and casual assessment or impression provided by office staff may help in distinguishing the troubled patient. Certain

[a] The Clevens Center for Facial Cosmetic Surgery and Imperial Spa, Merritt Island and Suntree, 1344 South Apollo Boulevard, Suite 100, Melbourne, FL 32901, USA
[b] University of Central Florida College of Medicine, Orlando, FL, USA
* The Clevens Center for Facial Cosmetic Surgery, 1344 South Apollo Boulevard, Suite 100, Melbourne, FL 32901, USA.
E-mail address: rossclevens@cfl.rr.com

Facial Plast Surg Clin N Am 17 (2009) 515–530
doi:10.1016/j.fsc.2009.06.005
1064-7406/09/$ – see front matter © 2009 Published by Elsevier Inc.

patients seem stable and pleasant with the physician, yet may be unreasonable or argumentative with ancillary staff. This may be a harbinger of trouble. If a trusted staff member expresses reservations regarding a potential patient's unfavorable behaviors or attitudes, then it is wise for the surgeon to heed this input.

As part of the overall assessment of the facelift patient, the surgeon may wish to consider medical and legal factors, such as prior surgery; history of litigation; or "doctor shoppers," patients having undergone an excessive number of cosmetic surgical procedures, ending up with an unaesthetic result, perhaps suggesting a body dysmorphic disorder.

Age

Age is an important consideration in facelift surgery. Because of the nature of the procedure, the patient population is shifted toward the more elderly. The overall vigor, attentiveness, and presentation of the aged patient should be considered. This evaluation includes not only the medical evaluation of the patient as discussed later, but other factors related to aging. This includes an assessment of the quality of the patient's skin, such as tissue elasticity, friability, bruisability, degree of solar damage, texture, and quality. This may adversely affect the vascularity and healing abilities of the patient. Generally, more fair complexed individuals have more favorable scarring, yet their incisions may stay pink much longer than a darker pigmented individual.

Becker and Castellano demonstrated that facelift surgery may be safely performed on American Society of Anesthesiologistis (ASA) class 1 and 2 patients older than age 75 years. This carefully selected, healthy, aged population does not experience a higher rate of complications or unfavorable outcomes as compared with a younger population.

In addition to considering the health status of the aging face patient, attention should also be turned toward the age and vigor of the primary caregiver. Because facelift is most commonly performed as an outpatient procedure, the postoperative care of the facelift patient may be relegated to a spouse, and the health status and wherewithal of this individual bears on the quality of care of the surgical patient. The vigor and ability of this other party should be informally assessed with respect to their capability to care for the facelift patient in the perioperative period.

Concurrent Medications in Facelift

Part of the history and physical examination of every surgical patient includes an inventory of the patient's current and recent medications including anticoagulants and steroids. Over-the-counter medications, vitamins, and occasional medications should also be evaluated. The patient's medication list provides insight into their general medical condition and appropriateness for rhytidectomy. Homeopathic remedies are remarkably common among aesthetic surgery patients. Often, patients neglect to consider or inform the surgeon of their concurrent use of vitamins, minerals, and herbal remedies. In general, the surgeon should consider advising the patient to discontinue the use of all homeopathic remedies for 10 to 14 days before surgery and 10 to 14 days subsequent to surgery. To minimize the risk of complications related to unknown vitamins and minerals, these broad recommendations mitigate the likelihood of a medication-related unfavorable result. Isotretinoin (Accutane) is associated with poor healing and increased scarring; the use of isotretinoin in low dose in middle aged and perimenopausal patients to control complexion is not uncommon and so should be considered even in the facelift patient age range. Facelift surgery should be delayed for 12 to 18 months following the cessation of Accutane therapy.

Cardiopulmonary Assessment for Facelift Surgery

As part of any medical evaluation, it is imperative to evaluate the patient's cardiac and pulmonary status. Hypertension is associated with a significantly increased risk of bleeding, bruising, and hematoma formation. Attentive perioperative control of hypertension is mandated. Of particular importance with respect to cardiac status, a functional assessment of cardiac condition, such as an exercise or nuclear stress test, may be indicated in instances of impaired cardiac performance. Patients with chronic obstructive pulmonary disease, for example, may have worsened cough and Valsalva associated with anesthesia and a lengthy procedure that may be associated with an increased risk of postoperative bleeding.

In most instances of active cardiac or pulmonary disease, preoperative medical clearance from the patient's personal physician or an appropriate internal medicine physician should be considered. The goal of the medical preoperative evaluation is to assess medical problems in surgical patients, to determine how best to manage these problems during surgery, and to provide recommendations for perioperative care. Preoperative risk assessment is based on two factors: the type of surgery to be performed and the patient's health.

Other Medical Considerations in Facelift Surgery

Patients with diabetes are particularly prone to bruising, delayed healing, infection, and displeasing scarring. Those with a history of alopecia may experience a greater degree of incisional alopecia than typical patients. Particular attention should be paid to the facial neurologic history and examination of the patient with query regarding Bell's palsy and trigeminal neuralgia. Patients with an immunocompromised status either of a primary or a secondary nature caused by other medications or disorders, such as rheumatologic disease, may experience infection and delayed healing.

The prospective facelift patient should be asked regarding their personal and family history of bleeding and clotting disorders. A family or personal history of bleeding or easy bruisability demands attention. A history of prolonged dysfunctional uterine bleeding, prior procedures complicated by hematoma, or difficulty with bleeding after dental extractions are concerning historical features. Prior radiation therapy may be associated with disrupted skin vascularity, diminished elasticity, and poor healing. Attention should be paid to the patient's skin type and ethnic heritage because this may be related to healing ability and scar resolution.

A review of the patient's anesthetic history is valuable. Patients should be questioned with respect to any personal or family history of significant complications related to the administration of anesthesia, such as malignant hyperthermia. Other historical facts, such as a personal tendency toward nausea and vomiting after anesthesia, assist in guiding the intraoperative anesthetic care of the patient and the postoperative management of the patient with regard to antiemetics. Patients who demonstrate a tendency toward motion sickness are more likely to experience postoperative nausea and vomiting; this information helps guide the anesthetic and postoperative care of the patient.

Contraindications to Facelift Surgery

Cigarette smoking is a relative contraindication to facelift surgery. Smoking is associated with a 12- to 20-fold increase in risk of flap slough (**Figs. 1** and **2**). Some have suggested that the risk of flap loss and poor scarring is minimized with certain deep plane facelift techniques where the vascularity of the skin is preserved. Patients should be instructed to discontinue smoking and nicotine products for 2 to 4 weeks before and subsequent to surgery. Nicotine-replacement products, such

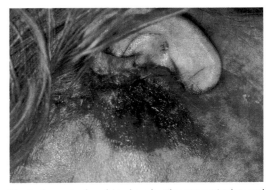

Fig. 1. Preauricular skin slough. The preauricular and postauricular regions represent the most distal segments of the facelift skin flap. These sites are prone to skin loss in smokers and in other instances where flap vascularity is compromised. (*Courtesy of* Shan R. Baker, MD, University of Michigan, Ann Arbor, MI.)

as nicotine patches, nicotine gum, nicotine nasal spray, and nicotine lozenges, are now widely available. Certain of these aids are now available over-the-counter, yet pose increased risks to the facelift patient. As already noted, patients may not

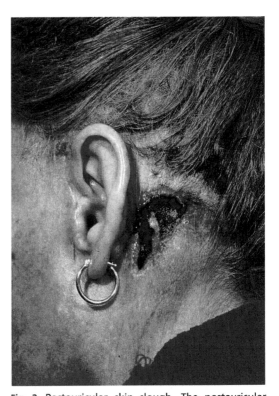

Fig. 2. Postauricular skin slough. The postauricular region is vulnerable to necrosis if the vascularity of the flap is insufficient. (*From* Baker SR. Rhytidectomy. In: Cummings CW, Flint PW, Harker LA, et al, editors. Cumming's otolaryngology head and neck surgery. 4th edition. Elsevier; 2005. p. 714–49.)

consider nonprescription medicines to be significant. Many smokers quit smoking around the time of surgery, yet switch to nicotine-containing products. The surgeon must consider this possibility because patients may either deny or neglect to mention the use of non–cigarette tobacco and nicotine products.

Prescription medications, such as bupropion SR (Zyban) and varenicline tartrate (Chantix), are non-nicotine pharmaceuticals that may assist patients to quit smoking before a facelift. Hypnotherapy or acupuncture may help some people quit smoking. Acupuncture involves placing extremely thin needles into the skin along specific acupuncture points to help curb the desire to smoke.

The current author has developed a separate consent form for current and former smokers, which details the risks of facial plastic surgery in the smoker. This consent form further requires the patient to attest that they have been tobacco and nicotine free for a minimum of 2 weeks before surgery and agree to remain so for at least 2 weeks subsequent to surgery. Notwithstanding these considerations, the current surgeon approaches such "tobacco-free" smokers with a modicum of trepidation and suspicion because smoking is a difficult addiction to cease without some degree of recidivism.

INTRAOPERATIVE CONCERNS IN FACELIFT SURGERY
Deep Venous Thrombosis Prophylaxis

Because of the typical prolonged length of the facelift procedure, patients are at a somewhat elevated risk of deep venous thrombosis. This is particularly magnified in patients with a heritable clotting disorder or history of prior lower-extremity deep venous thrombosis. Prevention of deep venous thrombosis through the use of prophylactic strategies is a noted recommendation in numerous clinical practice guidelines. Nonpharmacologic approaches include early mobilization of the patient postoperatively and the use of sequential intermittent pneumatic compression stockings. Pharmacologic approaches involve intraoperative anticoagulant therapy including the administration of subcutaneous unfractionated heparin, low-molecular-weight heparins, and heparinoids if there are no contraindications. Aspirin alone is not recommended as an agent to prevent deep venous thrombosis. Aspirin is relatively contraindicated in facelift surgery because of its tendency to promote postoperative bruising and bleeding. Deep venous thrombosis prophylaxis should be considered in facelift procedures, particularly those performed under general anesthesia. The present author uses thigh-high sequential compression stockings in all surgical procedures including facelift involving general anesthesia that lasts greater than 90 minutes.

Incisional Planning and Achieving Inconspicuous Scars

Patients are notably concerned regarding the scars that result from their surgery. Preoperative planning is required to achieve optimal cosmetic and functional results after making a skin incision. Patients are often misled to believe that there are no scars with facelift surgery. Patients should be reminded that once an incision is made, there is always a scar, but clinicians endeavor to create fine scars through inconspicuous incision placement and meticulous wound closure. Patients undergo facelifts to improve their facial appearance and do not consider visible or poor scarring an acceptable consequence (**Fig. 3**). It is important to have little to none of the telltale signs of having had a facelift, such as being pulled too tight or poor incisions resulting in conspicuous scars,

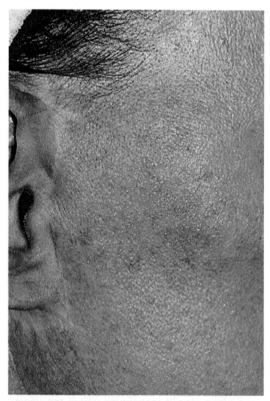

Fig. 3. Poor scarring following facelift surgery. This patient presented following facelift surgery with satisfactory results following her surgery in terms of facial contour. The patient was dissatisfied with obvious and noticeable incisions after her procedure.

loss of the sideburn hairline (**Fig. 4**), or an evident step-off behind the ear in the occipital hairline. To achieve the most favorable scars with facelift surgery, incisions should be carefully planned so as to minimize the alteration of the hairline pattern in both the male and female patient. This can be achieved by placing as many incisions as possible within hair-bearing regions. Sideburn-splitting incisions camouflage the temporal scar. Incisions within the occipital hair rather than along the occipital hairline similarly hide scars more favorably in the experience of the current author (**Fig. 5**). Incisions within non–hair-bearing skin should be crafted so as to lie within the contours of the periauricular region. Closure should be accomplished in a tension-free fashion. The closing of the wound should be performed in a meticulous and careful fashion with a multiple-layer closure. Minimal tension and multilayer closure minimize postoperative widening of the scar and anterior displacement of the tragus.

Hairline incisions are beveled parallel to hair follicles to avoid incisional alopecia. The postauricular limb of the incision should be placed on the

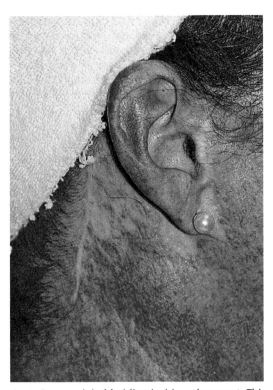

Fig. 5. Poor occipital hairline incision placement. This female patient has undergone facelift with an occipital hairline incision that is poorly positioned and associated with marked alopecia. Although this incision does not alter the position of the hairline, it may be more readily apparent in the female patient, especially if proper meticulous closure technique is not followed.

posterior surface of the ear because of its tendency to migrate posteriorly and inferiorly. Similarly, the retroauricular aspect of the facelift incision should be placed such that it crosses the mastoid non–hair-bearing region between the posterior surface of the ear and the hairline at a level corresponding to the widest horizontal aspect of the pinna. The scar passes from the superior aspect of the postauricular sulcus into the hairline in such a fashion that it crosses the shortest distance across the non–hair-bearing mastoid skin. With attentive placement of the scar in this region, the pinna itself also aids in camouflaging the scar. Additionally, this incision tends to migrate inferiorly, and high placement as described achieves a less conspicuous scar.

Many surgeons favor a retrotragal incision in women because this makes the scar discontinuous and arguably less apparent. Great care must be taken so as not to distort the shape or appearance of the tragus. A misshapen tragus or loss of the pretragal concavity is telltale sign of prior facelift surgery. Other surgeons prefer

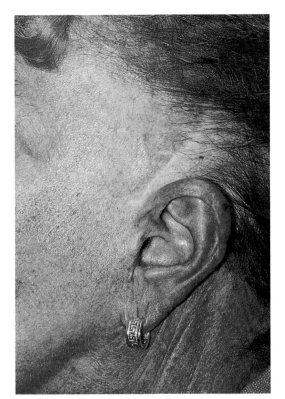

Fig. 4. Marked temporal hair loss. This patient suffers from severe alteration of the hairline, loss of the sideburn hair, and elevation of the temporal hairline. This deformity is avoidable with thoughtful incision planning and less dramatic pull of the skin.

a pretragal incision in women, believing that this is more favorable. The pretragal or retrotragal placement of the incision is generally left to individual surgeon's preference. In men, the incision is generally created in a pretragal fashion so as not to pull hair-bearing skin around the tragus and into the ear canal.

Avoiding Auricular Deformities

Anterior displacement of the tragus may be minimized by placing a stay suture anterior to the tragus that facilitates a tension-free closure minimizing pull of the skin in this region. This technique also contributes to recreating the natural pretragal depression. Careful replacement of the earlobe in a tension-free fashion contributes to avoiding the pixie ear deformity. Just as a stay suture may be placed in the pretragal region to facilitate in achieving a natural contour, so too may a tension-relieving suture be placed beneath the earlobe. Often, a bit of excess skin is left in this region to avoid tension. The incision around the earlobe is another potential visible area. Although the incision must be made at the junction of the earlobe and facial skin, the earlobe needs to be cradled after to keep this incision away from being ultimately seen. This technique almost always results in a more detached or separated earlobe from the side of the head, which must be closed with a few small sutures, but the facelift incision sits up high under the earlobe. Even if there is some inferior descent over time, it should remain inconspicuous and avoid the pixie ear deformity (**Fig. 6**).

The Safe Administration of Local Anesthesia

Local anesthesia with epinephrine is generally injected at the time of facelift surgery to facilitate hemostasis and postoperative patient comfort. The infiltration of local anesthesia is typically performed whether the procedure is being performed under general anesthesia, local anesthesia, or intravenous sedation. Whereas the anesthesiologist or anesthetist is responsible for the inhalational or intravenous anesthetic care of the patient, the surgeon bears responsibility for the injected local anesthesia. The surgeon must be aware of the limits of dosing of these medications (**Table 1**).

The maximum dose of lidocaine with epinephrine is on the order of 7 mg/kg; however, the maximum dose of plain lidocaine (without epinephrine) is only 3 to 5 mg/kg. Many surgeons elect to mix bupivacaine with lidocaine. The maximum dose of bupivacaine is 2.5 mg/kg. If lidocaine and bupivacaine are mixed, the relative

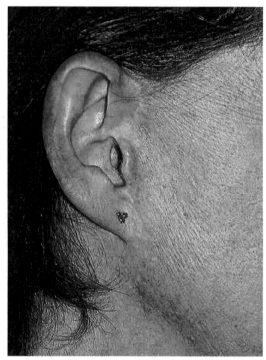

Fig. 6. Pixie ear deformity. Although the incisions in this patient have healed satisfactorily and are well-placed, the pixie ear deformity is noted. The ear lobule is unnaturally elongated as a result of an inferiorly directed tension on the ear lobule. This deformity may be avoided by closing the earlobe in a tension-free fashion.

contribution of the maximum dose of each local anesthetic must be calculated and taken into consideration to avoid complications related to local anesthetic. The maximum dose of epinephrine is 0.01 mg/kg with a maximum of 0.5 mg subcutaneously. The subcutaneous injection of local anesthesia is generally eliminated within 1.5 to 2 hours.

The most common source of complications related to local anesthesia is improper dosing. Inadvertent intravenous injection of local anesthetics during regional anesthesia can also result in potentially serious complications, such as seizures or cardiovascular collapse.

It is rarely considered, and perhaps not known to many surgeons, that on the induction of anesthesia and endotracheal intubation the anesthesiologist often administers an intubating dose of intravenous lidocaine on the order of 50 to 100 mg. This initial bolus dose must be considered in the surgeon's calculation of safe dosing.

In toxicity with local anesthetic in aesthetics, central nervous systems generally precede the cardiovascular symptoms. Neurologic signs

Table 1
Common local anesthetics

Generic Name	Concentration	Maximum Total Adult Dose	Lipid Solubility	Onset	Protein Binding	Duration of Effect
Lidocaine (Xylocaine)	1%–2%	4.5–5 mg/kg, not to exceed 300 mg	30 mL of 1%; 15 mL of 2%	<2 min	64%	30–60 min
Lidocaine with epinephrine	1%–2% lidocaine with epinephrine 1:100,000 or 1:200,000	7 mg/kg, not to exceed 500 mg	50 mL of 1%; 25 mL of 2%	<2 min	64%	30–60 min
Bupivacaine (Marcaine, Sensorcaine)	0.25%–50%	2.5 mg/kg, not to exceed 175 mg	70 mL of 0.25%; 35 mL of 0.5%	5 min	>95%	2–4 h
Bupivacaine with epinephrine	0.25% bupivacaine with epinephrine 1:200,000	3.5 mg/kg, not to exceed 225 mg	90 mL of 0.25%	5 min	>95%	4–7 h

include lightheadedness, dizziness, circumoral paresthesia, visual disturbances, altered vision, auditory disturbances, shivering, muscle twitching, tremors, and ultimately generalized-clonic convulsions. Under general anesthesia, the early signs of initial toxicity are often masked. The management of toxicity includes establishing or maintaining a safe airway with 100% oxygen administration. Convulsions should be treated with anticonvulsant drugs, such as thiopentone (150–200 mg IV) or diazepam (10–20 mg IV). Profound hypotension and bradyarrhythmias should be treated with an intravenous atropine (0.5–1.5 mg) in colloid or crystalloid infusions. Adrenaline may be required for severe hypotension or bradycardia.

Bupivacaine has a significant protein-bound component. Bupivacaine depresses the spontaneous pacemaker activity in the sinus node and exceeding the safe dose may result in sinus bradycardia, negative inotropy, and ultimately sinus arrest, which is very difficult to reverse because of the significant protein-bound component. In patients with ventricular fibrillation caused by bupivacaine toxicity, cardiopulmonary resuscitation should be continued and bretylium may facilitate cardioversion. Although bretylium tosylate injection is an antifibrillatory and antiarrhythmic agent, it is important to note that bretylium has been removed from some crash carts because it may no longer be part of the advanced cardiac life support (ACLS) protocol. Bupivacaine toxicity may be irreversible, and although common, its use should be prudent and carefully measured.

Technical Considerations in Suction-Assisted Lipectomy

The removal of excess or displaced fat from the cervicofacial region is often indicated during facelift to achieve a satisfactory contour of the neckline and jawline. Flap elevation is best achieved with pretunneling using liposuction cannulae that is not yet attached to suction. Liposuction is often used to sculpt the lower face and neck. Redundant fat may be removed through liposculpture throughout the jaw, submandibular, and submental regions. Liposuction is accomplished with small-diameter (1.5–3 mm) cannulae or wands. Ordinary operating room wall canister suction creates more than adequate negative pressure to achieve the desired effect. The use of a liposuction aspirator machine may predispose to contour irregularities because the negative pressure generated is too great for facial applications. During liposuction, the port of the cannula should be directed away from (rotated 180 degrees from) the undersurface of the skin to avoid dimpling.

Liposuction is best performed in a criss-cross section throughout a region with passes of the cannula directed at right angles to one another so as to achieve a smooth and uniform result. Closed cervicofacial liposuction may be performed through four access ports: one located superoposterior to each ear lobule and two situated at each lateral aspect of the submental crease. Through these four sites, the neck and submental regions may be accessed through two ports so that criss-cross liposuction may be achieved throughout. For example, the right neck is accessed through both the right submental incision and the right periauricular port so that the area is addressed from two directions achieving a smoother and more uniform result. In facelift surgery, this action facilitates flap elevation and then the areas may be reassessed under direct vision followed by open liposuction where necessary.

Nonetheless, the amount of fat to be removed is somewhat less than it seems on examination or might be anticipated even by the experienced facelift surgeon. The volume of fat removed is often just a few milliliters. A satisfactory degree of fat removal is accomplished making certain that an adequate thin layer of subcutaneous fat remains beneath the dermis. Overaggressive liposuction scars the dermis creating tethering in an unnatural contour and is associated with ridging and contour deformities (**Figs. 7** and **8**). Liposuction is often avoided superior to one finger breadth below the jawline; otherwise, inadvertent nerve injury to the marginal mandibular nerve may occur.

Avoiding Contour Irregularities in Facelift

Contour irregularities, such as dimpling, ridging, or the cobra deformity (hollowing in the submental region between the medial leaves of the sternocleidomastoid muscle) are often a result of irregular liposuction or overly aggressive liposuction. This may result from directing the port of the liposuction cannula toward the undersurface of the skin. The port should be directed away from (rotated 180 degrees from) the undersurface of the skin. Treatment of the irregularities or prevention of these irregularities emphasizes the importance of conservatism in fat removal.

Proper skin redrapage and closure are keys to preventing tethering and puckering of the skin. This is prevented through appropriate undermining of the skin in the region of closure so that the skin lies smooth and tension-free once it is replaced. The direction of lift should be posterior

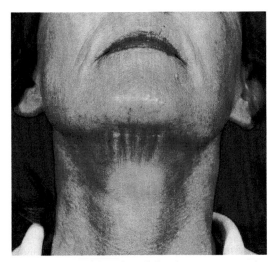

Fig. 7. Submental banding following overaggressive liposuction. Excessive fat removal or aggressive liposuction with scarification of the dermis may result in banding and an unnatural contour. This deformity is difficult to correct. Early in the postoperative period, massage and the judicious use of triamcinolone injections may help to minimize such irregularities. In the long run, the juxtaposition of soft tissue or fat grafting may diminish the appearance of banding. Avoidance of overaggressive lipocontouring is an important tenet. (*Courtesy of* Shan R. Baker, MD, University of Michigan, Ann Arbor, MI.)

along the mandible, yet superoposterior along the cheek. Failure to rotate and advance the flap in the proper vector may contribute to a stepped occipital hairline, loss of the sideburn, or the swoosh effect. These deformities are hallmarks of the conspicuous facelift. The swoosh effect is often seen with extensive skin undermining in conjunction with limited deeper dissection or forceful misdirected redrapage of the skin as seen in a skin-only lift. A stepped occipital hairline, loss

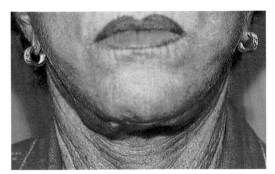

Fig. 8. Submental deformity after asymmetric neck contouring. Care must be taken at the time of surgery to contour the face and neck evenly at the time of facelift to avoid an unnatural appearance and telltale sign of prior poorly performed facelift surgery.

of the sideburn, and the swoosh effect are hallmarks of the conspicuous facelift.

Drains, if used, should generally be removed within 24 hours and certainly within 48 hours if possible to prevent subdermal irregularities. The use of a postoperative compression dressing further facilitates flap adhesion and eliminates dead space. This also may reduce the incidence of postoperative hematoma or seroma. It is important that the bandage is placed in a careful fashion so as to avoid excessive pressure, which may compromise the blood flow to the flaps creating pressure necrosis with the potential for scarring.

Treatment of contour abnormalities includes massage, judicious triamcinolone injections, and time. If these interventions fail over a 6- to 12-month period, then the surgeon may wish to consider fat grafting, reapproximation of the platysmal muscle, or resuspension of the skin flap; unfortunately, these approaches often meet limited success.

Flap Elevation to Preserve Vascular Supply

Flap elevation during facelift surgery should proceed within the subcutaneous plane. As noted, this may be performed or facilitated through the neck and submental region with a spatula cannula. The subdermal plexus vascularizes the skin. Regardless of flap elevation technique, care should be taken during development of the skin flap so as not to injure the subdermal plexus. Again, this is accomplished by preserving a layer of subcutaneous fat beneath the elevated skin.

As in reconstructive surgery, increasing flap length for a given width is also associated with decreasing vascular stability of the skin. Longer skin flaps undermined in the subcutaneous plane are associated with a more tenuous blood supply than a shorter length flap. A deep plane or sub–superficial musculoaponeurotic system dissection is associated with a shorter skin flap than a traditional skin lift. The richer blood supply of the multilayer sub–superficial musculoaponeurotic system or composite flap may improve viability of the skin. Some authors argue that this technique enhances flap viability, particularly in smokers. The most common area for skin necrosis or flap loss is typically the preauricular or postauricular skin. These sites represent the most distal segments of the flap and the weakest blood supply. The management of partial flap loss is typically conservative in management with limited debridement and the use of topical cleansing and antibiotic ointments.

Preserving Nerve Function in Facelift

Injury to the facial nerve is reported in 0.5% to 2.6% of patients. The most commonly injured branches are the frontal (**Fig. 9**) and marginal mandibular (**Fig. 10**) branches of the VII cranial nerve. The frontal branch is the most vulnerable of the branches because it has the fewest interconnections among other branches of the nerve.

The frontal or temporal branch of the facial nerve exits the parotid gland and runs within the superficial musculoaponeurotic system over the zygomatic arch into the temple region. The frontal branch enters the undersurface of the frontalis muscle and lies superficial to the deep temporalis fascia. To avoid injury to the frontal branch during elevation of facial flaps, the surgeon should elevate either in a subcutaneous plane or deep to the superficial musculoaponeurotic system. The frontal branch of the facial nerve is most commonly injured during elevation of the temporal portion of the facelift flap.

In the surgical position, the marginal mandibular nerve is found with the lowest point about 1 to 2 cm below the mandible between the posterior and anterior facial veins. The marginal branch lies deep to the platysma throughout much of its course. It becomes more superficial approximately 2 cm lateral to the corner of the mouth and ends on the undersurface of the muscles. The marginal mandibular nerve may be injured along the jawline and so flap elevation or liposuction should be reserved to one finger breadth or greater below the jawline in the submental region.

Sensory nerve injury is much less noticed in the aging face patient, although nearly 7% of patients

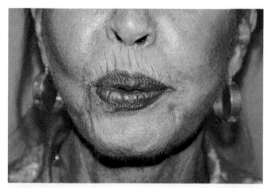

Fig. 10. Weakness of the marginal mandibular branch of the facial nerve. Note that the patient is having difficulty pursing her lips symmetrically, suggesting injury to the marginal mandibular branch of the facial nerve. (*Courtesy of* Shan R. Baker, MD, University of Michigan, Ann Arbor, MI.)

report some loss of sensation in the distribution of the great auricular nerve. The most common site of injury for the greater auricular nerve is in the region of the sternocleidomastoid muscle. The great auricular nerve lies deep to the superficial layer of the investing deep fascia as it ascends vertically over the sternocleidomastoid muscle. It divides into anterior and posterior branches to supply the periauricular region. The great auricular nerve is located 6 cm below the tragus at the anterior margin of the muscle to 9.5 cm below the tragus at the posterior margin of the muscle. Deep flap elevation in this region may create injury to the nerve and disruption of sensation in its distribution.

Vigilance Against Hematoma Formation in Facelift

Factors associated with hematoma may be divided into those attributes that are pre-existing, such as hypertension, pulmonary disease, cigarette smoking, diabetes, coagulation derangement, and male gender, as opposed to failure to achieve or recognize adequate hemostasis. Despite that all of these factors can be controlled and managed to some extent by the surgeon either by way of patient selection or medical management, hematomas nonetheless occur in the best of hands. Hematoma is an unfortunate postoperative complication of facelift that is seen in 1% to 15% of patients, although this number is more commonly cited in the 1.5% to 4% range in the hands of experienced surgeons. Expanding hematomas are observed with a twofold to fourfold increased relative risk in hypertensive patients, smokers, and in men. The etiology in hypertensive patients is believed to be an uncontrolled postoperative spike in blood pressure

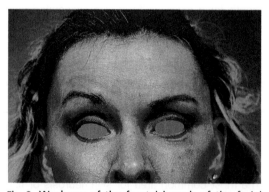

Fig. 9. Weakness of the frontal branch of the facial nerve. Observe that the patient is able to elevate her right brow, but not her left brow, suggesting injury to the left frontal branch of the facial nerve. (*From* Baker SR. Rhytidectomy. In: Cummings CW, Flint PW, Harker LA, et al, editors. Cumming's otolaryngology head and neck surgery. 4th edition. Elsevier; 2005. p. 714–49.)

leading to excessive bleeding. Smokers exhibit increased bruising, swelling, and often impaired blood supply and clotting accounting for the increased risk of hematoma seen in these patients. Men exhibit a higher incidence of hematoma formation because of the increased blood supply observed in the bearded skin of a male, and the increased activity level and lower degree of compliance witnessed in male, as compared with female, patients. Valsalva with increased venous pressure may be observed with coughing, retching caused by vomiting, or straining contributing to postoperative bleeding. A major or expanding hematoma is heralded by increasing pain, pressure, restlessness, or apprehension and often this may be sudden in onset after physical exertion (**Figs. 11** and **12**).

There are numerous operative strategies that may help prevent the occurrence of hematoma in the facelift patient. Appropriate preoperative preparation of the patient is critical, not only with respect to the management of hypertension, but also with respect to monitoring preoperative and postoperative medications including the elimination of blood thinners and homeopathic remedies for some time period, both before and subsequent to surgery. Notwithstanding medical management,

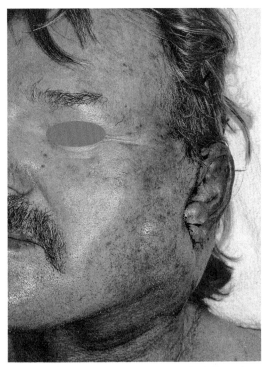

Fig. 12. Major expanding hematoma following facelift. This major hematoma recognized the evening of surgery required return to the operating room for evacuation. (*Courtesy of* Shan R. Baker, MD, University of Michigan, Ann Arbor, MI.)

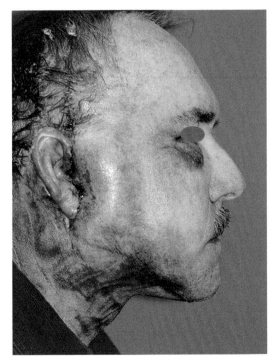

Fig. 11. Major hematoma following facelift. This major hematoma discovered on the first postoperative day necessitated operative evacuation. (*Courtesy of* Shan R. Baker, MD, University of Michigan, Ann Arbor, MI.)

there is no substitute for meticulous intraoperative hemostasis where the surgeon is certain that all intraoperative bleeding has ceased. The current author requests that his anesthesiologist maintain the patient normotensive or within 10% of baseline during the procedure. Blood pressure tends to drift below baseline with the administration of general anesthesia and so many anesthesiologists tend to manage the patient under general anesthesia with a somewhat lower than resting blood pressure, often with a systolic blood pressure 20 to 30 mm HG below baseline. This drop in systolic pressure may mask inadequate hemostasis. As a further precaution, this author instructs the anesthesiologist to raise the blood pressure 20 to 30 mm Hg above baseline before wound closure to observe for bleeding. This is accomplished by the anesthesiologist, who titrates the intravenous administration of phenylephrine or ephedrine under careful monitoring.

A shorter subcutaneous elevation combined with a deeper plane technique may reduce the risk of hematoma formation in virtue of creating less dead space. Suction drains and pressure dressings may also mitigate the risk of hematoma formation. Keen postoperative control of blood pressure, nausea, and vomiting help to prevent unwanted hypertensive episodes during the perioperative period. In some patients postoperative blood pressure management may be facilitated with the use of clonidine, 0.1 to 0.2 mg daily, for 3 to 5 days after surgery.

There are a number of tissue adhesives that facilitate flap adhesion and may aid in hemostasis, such as platelet-rich plasma, Tisseel, Surgifoam, FloSeal, and Plasmax. Platelet gel, also known as "platelet-rich plasma" or "platelet-enhanced leukocyte-rich gel," is a substance created by pheresing platelet-rich plasma from whole blood and combining it with thrombin and calcium or other activators to form a coagulum. This gel may facilitate hemostasis and flap adhesion. Tisseel is a two-component fibrin biomatrix that offers highly concentrated human fibrinogen to seal tissue and stop diffuse bleeding. Surgifoam is an absorbable gelatin sponge comprised of malleable, porcine gelatin absorbable sponge intended for hemostatic use by applying to a bleeding surface. FloSeal consists of a bovine-derived gelatin matrix component and thrombin that also functions as a hemostatic agent. The Plasmax system enables the creation of platelet-rich plasma and an autologous fibrin glue and sealant.

POSTOPERATIVE CONCERNS IN FACELIFT
Recognizing Hematoma

Major and expanding hematoma is heralded by increasing pain, pressure, restlessness, or apprehension and often this may be sudden in onset. The key to hematoma management lies with prevention and prompt treatment. An expanding cervical hematoma carries risks not only of poor and delayed healing, but also the potential for extrinsic airway compression if extensive. Treatment includes early recognition and hurried return to the operating room for evacuation under aseptic conditions. Before wound reclosure, the facelift bed is carefully inspected to ensure excellent hemostasis. Many of the same considerations noted previously to avoid hematoma at the time of initial surgery are also used at the time of evacuation of the hematoma to guard against reformation of the hematoma. Minor collections may be treated with needle aspiration and pressure dressings. Untreated hematoma may be further complicated by skin necrosis and scarring, infection, and unfavorable healing including contour deformities.

Managing Unfavorable Scars

Unfavorable scarring or hypertrophic scar formation is most commonly a result of excessive

tension, hematoma formation, or flap necrosis (**Fig. 13**). Other contributing factors include elevation of a skin flap that is too thin such that the subdermal plexus has been compromised, electrocautery on the undersurface of the skin, pressure necrosis from a bandage that has been too tight, clandestine use of tobacco or nicotine, and in diabetic or vasculopathic patients. The most vulnerable area for skin loss is found in the most distal and dependent segments of the flap, most frequently the post-auricular and temporal preauricular regions. Treatment for hypertrophic scar formation includes massage, the use of steroid-impregnated tape, triamcinolone injections, 5-fluorouracil injection, silicone gel and sheeting, and the passage of time. In the long run, unsatisfactory scars may require scar revision, dermabrasion, laser skin resurfacing, or 585-nm pulsed dye laser treatment. Earlobe distortion, known as the "pixie ear" or "devils ear" deformity, is

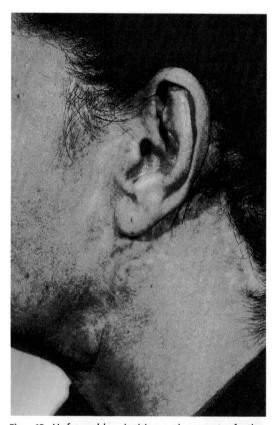

Fig. 13. Unfavorable incision placement further complicated by poor wound healing after facelift. This patient experienced thickened and hypertrophic scarring throughout her wounds. This unfavorable scarring is further highlighted because of poor and conspicuous incision placement.

caused by failure to inset the lobule properly, often with excessive inferior tension in this region. Repair of this deformity may be accomplished with a V toY technique.

Managing Hairline Changes in Facelift

Unfavorable hairline changes result from poor incisional planning. It is important to maintain the normal temporal and occipital hairlines and to plan for scars to settle hidden within the natural contours of the periauricular anatomy. Excessive subcutaneous undermining and improper flap drapage may contribute to disturbing the natural hairline. Camouflage of the disrupted hairline may be accomplished with an altered hairstyle, although this is often an unsatisfactory and displeasing option for the patient. Repair may be accomplished with the creation and rotation of local hair-bearing flaps or with hair replacement techniques. This is in contrast to alopecia, which may be transient in many patients for at least 6 to 8 weeks. Permanent alopecia is noted in 2% to 5% of patients. The most common etiology for this is excessive flap tension or failure to orient the incision properly relative to the hair follicle as noted previously. Treatment of alopecia may include triamcinolone injections, the topical application of minoxidil, scar revision to reapproximate hair-bearing skin to hair-bearing skin, and follicular hair transplant techniques.

Addressing the Dissatisfied Patient

Dissatisfied patients occur in the practice of even the most accomplished and experienced facial plastic surgeons. Patients elect to undergo aesthetic surgery to improve their self-image and appearance. The dissatisfied patient may result from a surgical complication; unrealistic patient expectations; or failure of the surgeon to inform the patient of the risks, benefits, and outcomes related to the procedure (**Fig. 14**). In addressing the dissatisfied patient, it is key to maintain the confidence of that patient. Listening carefully to the dissatisfied patient helps to foster a positive outlook. Accept the problems that the patient presents and schedule frequent supportive visits with the surgeon. Ancillary and aesthetic staff may be particularly helpful in connecting with a dissatisfied patient. Respond affirmatively and confidently to their concerns, but not defensively. It is important to recognize, for both the patient and the surgeon, that time improves many concerns. Finally, although it may be difficult for many surgeons to

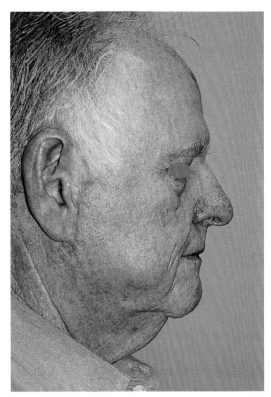

Fig. 14. The unfavorable result and dissatisfied patient. This well-educated engineer fell victim to the corporatized practice of medicine where a non-core physician performed a facelift procedure. This patient is disgruntled not only by the poor scars, but also by the abject lack of improvement in his facial contour and appearance following the procedure.

acknowledge their errors, offer revision surgery where indicated and necessary.

SUMMARY

Facelift is the stalwart procedure within the armamentarium of the aesthetic surgeon. Although there are numerous other procedures and techniques that aim to improve the appearance of the aging face, this important procedure remains key to the successful rejuvenation of the aging face. Facelift improves the appearance of the lower two thirds of the face and neck (**Fig. 15**). As with all surgical procedures, facelift is associated with certain risks and benefits. This article describes the sources of patient dissatisfaction and the avoidance and management of complications related to facelift surgery. A clinically oriented review that assists the practicing facial plastic surgeon in the avoidance, assessment, and management of complications encountered

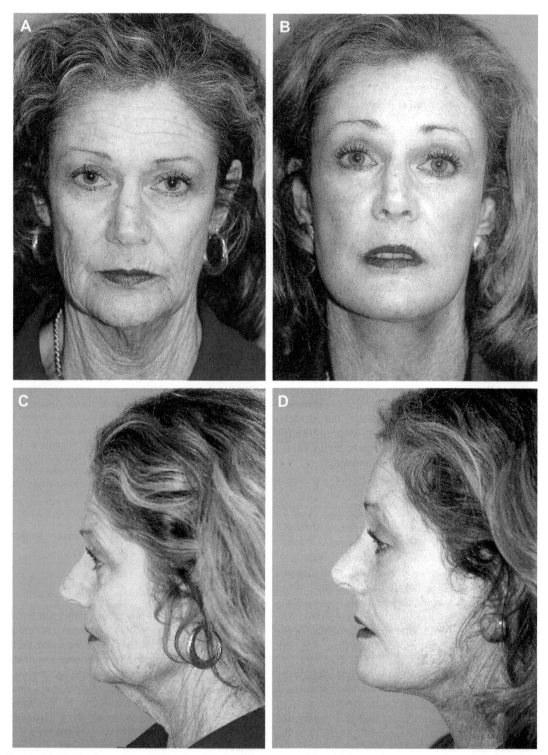

Fig. 15. (*A–D*) The favorable result following facelift surgery. This middle-aged woman is representative of the satisfied facelift patient who has enjoyed an uncomplicated postoperative course with natural rejuvenated facial contours and inconspicuous incisions.

during facelift surgery of the lower two thirds of the face and neck is offered.

ACKNOWLEDGMENT

The author expresses appreciation to Shan R. Baker, MD, University of Michigan Ann Arbor, for the use of certain images in this article. Some of these images may have appeared in Baker SR. Rhytidectomy. In: Cummings CW, Flint PW, Harker LA, et al, editors. Cumming's otolaryngology head and neck surgery. 4th edition. Elsevier; 2005. pp. 714–49; and Moyer J, Baker SR. Complications of rhytidectomy. Facial Plast Surg Clin North Am 13:469–478.

SUGGESTED READINGS

Adamson PA, Moran ML. Complications of cervicofacial rhytidectomy. Facial Plast Surg Clin North Am 1993;1:257–71.

Ash TF, Pruzinsky T. Body image: development and change. New York: Guilford Press; 1990.

Baker DC. Complications of cervicofacial rhytidectomy. Clin Plast Surg 1983;10:543–62.

Baker DC, Conley J. Avoiding facial nerve injuries in rhytidectomy. Plast Reconstr Surg 1979a;64:666–9.

Baker DV, Conley J. Avoiding facial nerve injuries in rhytidectomy: anatomical variations and pitfalls. Plast Reconstr Surg 1979b;964:781–95.

Baker SR. Rhytidectomy. Ch 30. In: Cummings CW, Flint PW, Harker LA, editors. 4th edition, Cumming's otolaryngology head and neck surgery, vol. 1. Philadelphia, Mosby: Elsevier; 2005. p. 714–49.

Becker FF. The preauricular portion of the rhytidectomy incision. Arch Otolaryngol Head Neck Surg 1994;120:166–71.

Beekhuis GJ. Facelift: postoperative hematoma, prevention and management. Laryngoscope 1980;90:164–7.

Berner RE, Morain WD, Noe JM. Postoperative hypertension as an etiological factor in hematoma after rhytidectomy: prevention with chlorpromazine. Plast Reconstr Surg 1976;57:314–9.

Burgess LP, Casler JD, Kryzer TC. Wound tension in rhytidectomy: effects of skin-flap undermining and superficial musculoaponeurotic system suspension. Arch Otolaryngol Head Neck Surg 1993;119:173–6.

Chang LD. Cigarette smoking, plastic surgery, and microsurgery. J Reconstr Microsurg 1996;12:467–74.

Cohen SR, Webster RC. Primary rhytidectomy: complications of the procedure and anesthetic. Laryngoscope 1983;93:654–6.

Daane SP, Owsley JQ. Incidence of cervical branch injury with marginal mandibular nerve pseudoparalysis in patients undergoing face lift. Plast Reconstr Surg 2003;11:2414–8.

Edgerton MT, Webb WL, Slaughter R, et al. Surgical results and psychosocial changes following rhytidectomy. Plast Reconstr Surg 1964;33:503–21.

Ellenbogen R. Avoiding visual tipoffs to face lift surgery: a troubleshooting guide. Clin Plast Surg 1992;19:447–54.

Ellenbogen R. Pseudoparalysis of the mandibular branch of the facial nerve after platysmal face-lift operation. Plast Reconstr Surg 1979;63:364–8.

Goin JM, Goin MK. Changing the body: psychological effects of plastic surgery. Baltimore (MD): Williams & Wilkins; 1981.

Goldwyn RM. Late bleeding after rhytidectomy from injury to the superficial temporal vessels. Plast Reconstr Surg 1991a;88:443–5.

Goldwyn RM. Late bleeding from superficial temporal vessels after rhytidectomy. Plast Reconstr Surg 1991b;88:443–5.

Hetter G. Lipoplasty: the theory and practice of blunt suction lipectomy. 2nd edition. Boston: Little Brown; 1990.

Hoffman S, Simon BE. Complications of submental lipectomy. Plast Reconstr Surg 1977;60:889–94.

Izquierdo R, Parry SW, Boydell CL, et al. The great auricular nerve revisited: pertinent anatomy for SMAS-platysma rhytidectomy. Ann Plast Surg 1991;27:44–8.

Kamer FM, Minoli J. Postoperative platysmal band deformity: a pitfall of submental liposuction. Arch Otolaryngol Head Neck Surg 1993;119:193–6.

Knize DM. The forehead and temporal fossa. New York: Lippincott, Williams & Wilkins; 2001.

Larrabee WF, Makielski KH, Henderson JL. Surgical anatomy of the face. 2nd edition. New York: Lippincott, Williams & Wilkins; 2004.

Lawson W, Naidu RK. The male facelift: an analysis of 115 cases. Arch Otolaryngol Head Neck Surg 1993;119:535–9.

Liebman EP, Webster RC, Gaul JR, et al. The marginal mandibular nerve in rhytidectomy and liposuction surgery. Arch Otolaryngol Head Neck Surg 1988;114:179–81.

Marten TJ. Facelift planning and technique. Clin Plast Surg 1997;24:269–308.

McKinney P. Prevention of injury to the great auricular nerve during rhytidectomy. Plast Reconstr Surg 1980;66:675–9.

McKinney P, Giese S, Placik O. Management of the ear in rhytidectomy. Plast Reconstr surg 1993;92:858–66.

Moffat DA, Ramsden RT. The deformity produced by a palsy of the marginal mandibular branch of the facial nerve. J Laryngol Otol 1977;91:401–10.

Moyer J, Baker S. Complications of rhytidectomy. Facial Plastic Surgery Clinics of North America 2005;13(3): 469–78.

Nason RW, Binahmed A, Torchia MG. Thliversis: clinical observations of the anatomy and function of the marginal mandibular nerve. Int J Oral Maxillofac Surg 2007;36:712–5.

Perkins SW, Williams JD, Macdonald K, et al. Prevention of seromas and hematomas after face-lift surgery with the use of postoperative vacuum drain. Arch Orolaryngol Head Neck Surg 1997; 123:743–5.

Rao VK, Morrison WA, O'Brien BM. Effect of nicotine on blood flow and patency of experimental microvascular anastomosis. Ann Plast Surg 1983;11:206–9.

Rees TD, Lee YC, Coburn RJ. Expanding hematoma after rhytidectomy: a retrospective study. Plast Reconstr Surg 1973;51:149–53.

Rees TD, Liverett DM, Guy CL. The effect of cigarette smoking on skin-flap survival in the face-lift patient. Plast Reconstr Surg 1984;73:911–5.

Riefkohl R, Wolfe JA, Cox EB, et al. Association between cutaneousocclusive vascular disease, cigarette smoking, and skin slough after rhytidectomy. Plast Reconstr Surg 1986;77:592–5.

Seckel BR. Facial danger zones. St Louis (MO): Quality Medical Publishing; 1994.

Webster RC, Kazda G, Hamdan US, et al. Cigarette smoking and face lift: conservative versus wide undermining. Plast Reconstr Surg 1986;77:596–604.

Management of Anesthesia and Facility in Facelift Surgery

Stephen Prendiville, MD*, Seth Weiser, CRNA

KEYWORDS

- Anesthesia • Facelift • Intravenous sedation
- Postoperative nausea/vomiting • Facial plastic surgery

The primary goal of elective cosmetic facial surgery is to achieve objective changes that are aesthetically pleasing; however, equally important is the patient's subjective assessment of the result and the process that lead to it. A safe, uneventful anesthetic helps keep a patient focused, prevents sequelae that can significantly prolong the healing period, and maintains a positive perception of the experience. One of the greatest sources of preoperative anxiety for a patient considering facial plastic surgery is the method and course of anesthesia. The purpose of anesthesia is to provide analgesia, amnesia, and a quiet and stable surgical field. Ideal anesthesia should achieve all these goals and allow a smooth transition into the postoperative phase without undue problems such as postoperative nausea/vomiting (PONV), prolonged sedation, or cardiovascular complications. This scenario allows the patient to think about recovery in a positive manner. The experience should be viewed in its entirety, from the process that brings the patient to the operating room, to the intraoperative course, and finally to a smooth and uneventful recovery.

Most cases performed in the senior author's facility are done so under propofol-based deep intravenous anesthesia with local anesthesia infiltration. The rational for preparation, choices of medication, intraoperative monitoring, and safety measures are explained in the following sections.

PREOPERATIVE PREPARATION AND SCREENING

In any surgical endeavor, the primary concern to patient and surgeon alike is safety. A significant portion of facial plastic and reconstructive surgery is elective, and the general expectation of American society is that lifestyle-enhancing elective plastic surgical procedures should be free of complications. Although patients must be informed that complications can and do occur, minimization of perioperative events is essential to build and maintain a successful practice. Ensuring a low perioperative morbidity begins with preoperative screening, assessment of risk, and preoperative clearance. Good anesthesia relies on good patient selection by the surgeon and on good judgment by the certified registered nurse anesthetist (CRNA)/anesthesiologist in monitoring the patient intraoperatively. The following guidelines are used in patient selection in the senior author's practice.

A thorough personal medical history and history of family bleeding tendencies should be recorded. A history of bruising, heavy menstrual periods, and frequent epistaxis should be pursued with appropriate laboratory testing (serum coagulation studies, platelet count, and von Willebrand's factor level, if necessary). The patient's entire medication history should be reviewed, and the patient should be asked directly about the use of dietary supplements, weight-loss aids, cocaine/illicit drugs, and oral isotretinoin and about recent bacterial cultures and/or antibiotic history. A special note should be made about the antibiotic history, given the increasing prevalence of community-acquired bacteria in many communities. Likewise, the medical history should elicit any and all medications that can contribute to decreased platelet clumping activity and/or coagulation cascade

9407 Cypress Lake Drive, Suite A, Fort Myers, Sarasota, FL 33919, USA
* Corresponding author.
E-mail address: steveprendiville@msn.com (S. Prendiville).

Facial Plast Surg Clin N Am 17 (2009) 531–538
doi:10.1016/j.fsc.2009.06.010
1064-7406/09/$ – see front matter © 2009 Elsevier Inc. All rights reserved.

dysfunction. This information includes a review of all nonsteroidal anti-inflammatory medications and herbal supplements (eg, gingko, echinacea, St John's wort). The use of nonsteroidal anti-inflammatory medications, herbal supplements, and vitamins (excluding multivitamins) is stopped at least 2 weeks before surgery; the use of aspirin is stopped at least 3 weeks before surgery. It is particularly important to discontinue aspirin, because it permanently acetylates the cyclo-oxygenase enzyme on the platelet and permanently affects an individual platelet's ability to bind to other platelets. Because the life cycle of the platelet is 90 days, a certain degree of platelet clotting dysfunction remains even after prolonged discontinuation. The questioning about the patient's previous anesthetic experiences should include a direct question about PONV. If the patient experienced difficulty and/or an adverse event, a review of the anesthesia record is advisable. In the senior author's practice, the patient routinely is called by the CRNA to obtain further details and to provide reassurance the night before surgery. A specific question about family history pertaining to malignant hyperthermia also should be included. Last, possible drug and/or latex allergies are reviewed.

A risk-assessment classification system was devised by the American Society of Anesthesiologists (ASA). The overwhelming majority of patients undergoing elective cosmetic surgical procedures should be ASA class I or II.

ASA I: Healthy individuals who have no systemic disease.

ASA II: Individuals who have one-system, well-controlled disease that does not affect daily activities. Smoking, obesity, and heavy alcohol use qualify an individual as ASA II.

ASA III: Individuals who have multisystem disease or well-controlled major system disease. The disease status limits daily activity.

ASA IV: Individuals who have severe incapacitating disease.

ASA V: Patient in imminent danger of death.

All patients, regardless of age, are required to have a preoperative complete blood cell count; all premenopausal women should be questioned about possible pregnancy and are required to take a preoperative urine pregnancy test on the morning of the procedure. All patients over 50 years of age are required to have an EKG, complete blood cell count, and serum electrolytes (within 30 days of the procedure). All patients who have chronic, stable cardiovascular diagnoses are required to see an internist or cardiologist for preoperative clearance. All patients taking any form of diuretic are required to have serum electrolytes to ensure that serum potassium is not marginally or severely depleted.

All patients are required to take nothing by mouth for at least 8 hours before the procedure (with the exception of medications taken with sips of water). This restriction generally requires no food or drink after midnight before the procedure. Patients are asked to maintain normal diet and hydration up to this point, however, because it is best to avoid taking a dehydrated, hypovolemic patient to the operating room.

All surgical and anesthesia consents are signed several days before the procedure. Last-minute changes or additions to the surgical procedure are strongly discouraged unless discussed during initial or subsequent consultations. Changes cannot be made to the consent if the patient has taken diazepam.

MONITORING EQUIPMENT/OPERATING ROOM SET-UP

Ultimately, successful anesthesia is a combination of a competent practitioner using good judgment and technique and appropriate, well-maintained equipment. In the state of Florida, most elective cosmetic surgical cases are performed in an outpatient surgery center (certified by the agency for health care administration (AHCA) or joint commission), or office-based surgical centers (accredited by the American Association for Accreditation of Ambulatory Surgical Facilities [AAAASF], the Accreditation Association for Ambulatory Health Care, or the joint commission or Florida state certified). The senior author's practice uses the latter option, with AAAASF certification. Certification requires a number of crucial pieces of equipment and safety devices: a crash cart containing all the medications required in each of the cardiac arrest and arrhythmia protocols and in malignant hyperthermia protocols; a defibrillator and/or automated external defibrillator; a patient monitor with oxygen saturation, heart rate, automated blood pressure capabilities and with optional end tidal CO_2/inhalational agent monitoring capability; a back-up power supply; a suction pump; and an anesthesia machine with vaporizer (if general anesthesia is to be used in the facility) (**Fig. 1**).

PATIENT SAFETY AND AIRWAY CONSIDERATIONS

One of the most common serious complications of surgical procedures relates to venous stasis and deep venous thrombosis (DVT). Individuals who are exposed to prolonged immobility for any

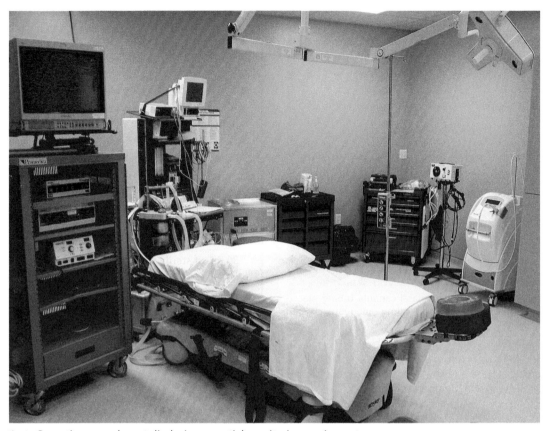

Fig. 1. Operating room layout displaying essential monitoring equipment.

reason are at increased risk for DVT. Women taking oral contraceptives, smokers, and individuals who have hypercoagulable states are at even higher risk. An obvious and potentially fatal consequence of DVT is pulmonary embolus. For this reason, venous stasis must be treated seriously, and its prevention must be built into the perioperative regimen of any surgical center. All patients undergoing intravenous sedation or general anesthesia in the senior author's facility are required to wear knee-high compression stockings, placed in the preoperative area. The patient then is asked to walk to the operating room to maintain venous return. Before induction of anesthesia, sequential compression devices (SCDs) are placed on the lower extremities to promote flow of blood in the legs and avoid venous stasis. It is critical to apply these devices before the induction of anesthesia, when the most profound vasodilatation and venous pooling are likely to occur. To make sure that compression is occurring when most needed, the SCDs are placed and activated in the operating room before placement of the intravenous line.

Maintenance of an adequate airway and sufficient oxygenation is crucial to patient safety. Airway management problems after induction of anesthesia are responsible for a very large percentage (50%–75%) of cardiac arrests in surgical cases.[1] For intravenous sedation, an oral airway is placed with a unique modification devised by the senior author (**Fig. 2**): (1) the nasal prongs are removed from a nasal cannula; (2) one section of the tubing is tied off; (3) the open section of tubing is threaded sequentially through the fenestrations in the central portion of the airway until the end of the oxygen delivery tube sits at the distal end of the oral airway; (4) the tubing is secured to the proximal oral airway with a rubber band. This device allows adequate airway maintenance and facilitates oxygenation (**Fig. 3**). Another option for maintaining an airway during deep sedation is the use of a laryngeal mask airway (LMA). LMAs tend to be somewhat bulky for facial surgery, however, and are rarely used in the senior author's practice. A dedicated sterilized instrument tray is maintained for tracheotomy in the case of true airway emergencies.

To avoid confusion, a written table is posted explaining how local anesthetics are to be mixed (**Box 1**), and this task is assigned to the same individual (a registered nurse) to provide consistency

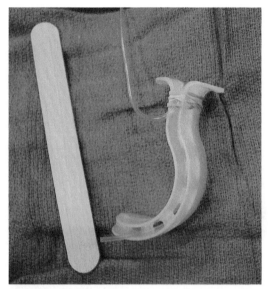

Fig. 2. Oral airway with nasal cannula tubing placed through fenestrations to allow adequate oxygen delivery.

and to prevent errors. An explanation of toxicity is provided, and a review of toxicities is required for all personnel in the operating room.

LOCAL ANESTHESIA

Local anesthetics are a cornerstone of facial plastic surgery; understanding their benefits and pitfalls is critical to successful patient management. Local anesthetic agents work by inhibiting nerve conduction via blockade of sodium channels in electrically excitable membranes.[2] These agents can be used as the sole form of analgesia/anesthetic via local infiltration or regional blocks or to supplement analgesia for a surgical field with intravenous sedation or general

| Box 1 |
| Solutions for facelift anesthesia |

Facelift Solution 1 (makes a 1:100,000 solution of local anesthetic with epinephrine)

25 mL of 1% lidocaine (250 mg lidocaine)

10 mL of 0.25% bupivacaine (25 mg Marcaine)

15 mL of sterile saline solution

0.5 mL of 1 mg/mL epinephrine (1:1000)

Facelift Solution 2 (makes a 1:100,000 solution of local anesthetic with epinephrine)

10 mL of 1% lidocaine (150 mg lidocaine)

10 mL of 0.25% bupivacaine (25 mg Marcaine)

30 mL of sterile saline solution

0.5 mL of 1 mg/mL epinephrine (1:1000)

Attention:

Toxicity for lidocaine with epinephrine is 7 mg/kg based on intravenous studies (for a healthy 70 kg-person, 490 mg or 49 mL of 1% lidocaine). Over the course of a 4-hour case, much of the lidocaine (half-life 1.5 h) initially infused will be metabolized.

Toxicity for bupivacaine (Marcaine, half-life of 4–6 hours) without epinephrine is 175 mg (70 mL of 0.25% Marcaine) per dose or 400 mg (160 mL of 0.25% Marcaine) over 24 h. The toxicity with epinephrine is 225 mg per dose (90 mL of 0.25% Marcaine). Marcaine toxicity is much more severe than lidocaine toxicity, and every effort should be made to keep Marcaine doses as low as possible.

anesthesia. Local anesthesia also can be administered in topical form using commercially available agents (EMLA) or special pharmacy-compounded agents to provide analgesia. Local anesthetics provide a reversible neural blockade by inhibiting or impeding impulse transmission in peripheral nerves or nerve endings. A non-depolarizing blockade occurs at the surface membrane of tissue cells such as nerve fibers and smooth and striated muscle. There are three main types of nerve fibers: A, B, and C.[3]

A. fibers are myelinated somatic nerves and are subclassified into alpha, beta, gamma, and delta categories. The alpha fibers are the largest and most rapidly conducting subgroup. The delta fibers are smallest and slowest.

B. fibers are myelinated, autonomic, preganglionic fibers.

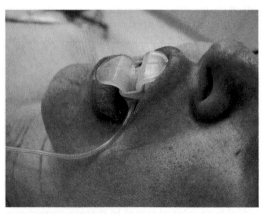

Fig. 3. Oral airway in place.

C. fibers are nonmyelinated somatic and auto-nomic small nerve fibers that are easily blocked.

Large A fibers (alpha and beta) convey motor function, proprioception, and touch. Small A fibers (gamma and delta) and C fibers subserve pain and temperature. The smaller fibers are easier to block and recover their function more rapidly than the larger nerve fibers.

Most clinically relevant local anesthetics are tertiary amines and are weak bases (pH 7–10). The more alkaline the local anesthetic solution, the more rapid is the onset of and effectiveness of the block. The pH of lidocaine accounts for its rapidity in onset and discomfort on injection. Because of the slightly alkaline nature of local anes-thetics, injection into an area of tissue inflammation (low pH, acidic environment) will reduce liberation of the free anesthetic base and diminish efficacy.

Lidocaine

Lidocaine is an amide-linked local anesthetic and is one of the most widely used anesthetics in facial plastic surgery. It is metabolized by the liver (cyto-chrome P450) and has a half-life of 1.5 to 2 h. When used intravenously, lidocaine also has anti-arrhythmic effects and central nervous effects such as amnesia and drowsiness. The potential for cardiac and central nervous system toxicity of intravenous lidocaine is indisputable, but there is some debate about the applicability of the toxic doses to subcutaneous injections as opposed to intravascular injections.[4] The toxic dose of lidocaine without epinephrine is listed as 3 to 5 mg/kg, and that of lidocaine with epinephrine is listed as 5 to 7 mg/kg. In many clinical situations, the senior author favors the use of lidocaine with 1:100,000 epinephrine, because the local vasoconstriction caused by the epinephrine (which is used for intra-operative hemostasis) allows greater duration of the anesthetic. One percent lidocaine contains 10 mg/mL. Therefore, for a healthy 70-kg person, the toxic dose of 1% lidocaine with 1:100,000 epinephrine is 490 mg or 49 mL (using the higher end of the toxicity scale). Whenever the injection has a high likelihood of becoming intravascular, the lower end of the toxicity scale is adhered to. In situations in which larger volumes of local anesthetic are used (eg, rhytidectomy), the lidocaine is diluted, using a consistent formula (see **Box 1**) to avoid issues of toxicity.

Bupivacaine

Bupivacaine is a stable, long-acting, highly protein-bound, highly lipid-soluble, amide-linked local anesthetic. It is metabolized primarily by the liver and has a half-life of 3.5 to 4 h. The toxic dose of bupivacaine is 2 to 2.5 mg/kg per dose or 400 mg over 24 h. The toxic dose for a healthy 70-kg person is 175 mg or 70 mL of 0.25% bupiva-caine. Bupivacaine toxicity (complete atrioventric-ular block, seizures) is difficult to reverse and is potentially lethal. Therefore, special care is taken to ensure that safe levels of bupivacaine are administered. For this reason, bupivacaine is used in the senior author's practice only for longer cases and with specific dilutions (see **Box 1**).

Cocaine

Cocaine is the only local anesthetic that possesses vasoconstrictive and local anesthetic properties. An ester-linked local anesthetic, it is not widely used in isolated facelift surgery. Toxicity is primarily cardiovascular, but neurotoxicity can occur. The toxic dose of cocaine is considered to be 4 mg/kg. Vials of topical cocaine for use in rhinoplasty or other nasal procedures contain 5 mL of 4% cocaine (200 mg). Communication between the surgeon and anesthesiologist or CRNA is essential before the administration of topical cocaine to allow for appro-priate responses to changes in heart rate and/or blood pressure that may ensue.

ANESTHETIC AGENTS
Inhalational Anesthesia

Most currently used inhalational agents are haloge-nated anesthetic drugs. This class of drugs includes isoflurane, desflurane, and sevoflurane (halothane and enflurane also are in this class but are used rarely). The inhalational agent most commonly used in the senior author's practice is sevoflurane because of its rapidity of induction, rapid recovery, easy control of anesthesia depth, and lower incidence of inhalational "hangover."[5] Sevoflurane is less soluble than older anesthetic agents and achieves a higher partial pressure in the brain during induction. Likewise, the fall in partial pressure is equally rapid when administra-tion is stopped, allowing a quicker recovery. Sevo-flurane also is less irritating to the airway during induction.[2] Sevoflurane is more expensive than other inhalational agents, however, and it has an active metabolite known as "compound A" (more commonly found with closed loop anesthesia and low flows) that is potentially nephrotoxic. Desflur-ane offers several of the advantages of sevoflurane but tends to be more irritating to the airway and has a higher incidence of laryngospasm.

Intravenous Agents

Propofol is the newest of the intravenous agents to be introduced (1984). Propofol's mechanism of action is via initiation of hypnosis; it can be used both as an inducing agent and for maintenance of anesthesia. It is metabolized by the liver and is excreted in the urine; its half-life is 3 to 12 h. The benefits of propofol are the rapidity of onset and ease of anesthesia maintenance with continuous infusion, without the drawbacks of nausea or drug hangover.[2] Propofol should be avoided in patients who have known sensitivity to egg lecithin.

Benzodiazepenes have been used for many years as anxiolytics and as adjuvant agents for induction of anesthesia. The most commonly used drug from this class is intravenous midazolam, which has rapid onset, enhances gamma-aminobutyric acid effects, and induces anterograde amnesia. It is metabolized by the liver and is excreted in the urine.

Narcotics also are old stand-bys for intravenous sedation and analgesia. The most commonly used narcotic in the senior author's practice is fentanyl, a synthetic opioid agonist, that is metabolized by the liver and is excreted in the urine. The potential for nausea with administration of narcotics is well known, and every effort is made to reduce the amount of fentanyl given.

MANAGEMENT OF PERIOPERATIVE HYPERTENSION IN FACELIFT SURGERY

There are various opinions about the most appropriate method of managing blood pressure in facial plastic surgical cases. Although the method of management depends somewhat on the individual patient's physiology, the consensus seems to be that blood pressure should be kept at or near the low end of normotension for the individual patient. If a healthy patient's blood pressure is 115 to 120 mm Hg systolic under everyday conditions, the senior author would like the patient's blood pressure to be at 90 to 100 mm Hg systolic (or 15 to 20 points below the preoperative starting point) while under anesthesia. A patient with a starting point of 85 to 90 mm Hg systolic, however, is better kept within the natural range. Careful monitoring of heart rate is essential because hypotension accompanied by tachycardia may signal hypovolemia. Oral clonidine is administered routinely in the preoperative area to initiate normotension unless the preoperative blood pressure dictates otherwise.

During times of intense stimulation (intubation, initial injection of local anesthesia, or alternatively, when local anesthetia at the point of dissection may be inadequate), one should expect elevated blood pressures and tachycardia; this condition may be transient and should be treated if only it persists. As an operation progresses, inadequate local analgesia should be ruled out as the cause of blood pressure changes before other measures are pursued. Injection of local anesthesia can be painful, and spikes in blood pressure and pulse are to be expected. Again, it is very important to avoid over-zealous treatment of such hemodynamic spikes. Should the blood pressure elevation not improve significantly in several minutes, the following algorithm is used: (1) If the heart rate is also elevated, first administer a small dose of propanolol (a nonselective beta-blocker). An initial dose of 0.25 mg is given intravenously and is repeated once after a few minutes if the first dose does not remedy the situation. (2) If the blood pressure is not responsive, 2.5 mg of hydralazine (an alpha blocker) is given intravenously. This dose can be repeated in 15 minutes if needed (to a maximum of three doses). Usually this treatment will last for the duration of the surgery and also will provide a smooth postoperative course. The senior author tends to avoid labetalol (a selective alpha-1 blocker and a nonselective beta blocker) because of its short duration and the potential for postoperative orthostatic hypotension in ambulatory patients. If labetalol is administered, a small test dose (2 mg intravenously) should be administered to assess the patient's initial response. A large bolus of labetalol (10 mg) in a patient who has not previously received the drug or who is hypovolemic could place the patient in a far worse situation.

During general anesthesia for rhinoplasty the agent of choice is sevoflurane. The senior author rarely paralyzes patients for this procedure; the ultimate goal is to have the patient breathe spontaneously throughout the case while titrating in small doses of fentanyl to reduce the dose of sevoflurane required. When general anesthesia is used, an oral Rae tube either is taped to the lower jaw or is tied with dental floss to the upper incisor. An LMA also is an option but can be very cumbersome.

PREVENTING POSTOPERATIVE NAUSEA
Prevention

One of the most vexing and potentially most costly postanesthesia problems for patient and surgeon alike is PONV. A patient who experiences PONV is more likely to have postoperative problems such as hematoma after rhytidectomy, epistaxis after rhinoplasty, or prolonged edema/ecchymosis after blepharoplasty. Therefore, prevention of PONV should be addressed directly in the perioperative management of the patient. Should the problem arise, aggressive management is suggested. Prevention begins with preoperative education of the patient about narcotic-associated nausea. In the absence of a wound complication, most facial plastic surgical cases are not associated with severe pain. Patients are educated about the nature of discomfort they may experience. For example, rhytidectomy patients are informed about tight dressings, and rhinoplasty patients are educated about the inability to breathe nasally with the presence of nasal packing. All patients are given prescriptions for propoxyphene in the event of postoperative discomfort, but patients and their care givers are instructed to use acetaminophen as the first-line agent for pain and oral diazepam as the first-line agent for anxiety. Intraoperatively, dexamethasone is administered to minimize edema and for its antiemetic properties.

Patients are given a prescription for two 40-mg tablets of aprepitant (Emend). The patient is instructed to take one of the tablets on the morning of surgery with a sip of water; the other tablet is reserved for possible PONV. Aprepitant selectively antagonizes substance P/neurokinin 1 receptors and is a very potent antiemetic agent used for patients receiving chemotherapy. It is more expensive than most other antiemetic options. Ondansetron (a 5-HT3 receptor antagonist), 4 mg ODT, is a second-line antiemetic option if the patient is unable to obtain aprepitant. Similar dosing instructions are given.

Active Postoperative Nausea

Any patient complaining of PONV in the recovery room is given ondansetron, 4 mg intravenously; this dose is repeated in 30 minutes if nausea persists. Patients who have a history of PONV, patients undergoing brow lift procedures, patients who have a history of migraines, and patients scheduled to undergo lengthy procedures are given an additional prescription for 25-mg prochlorperazine suppositories (to antagonize dopamine D2 receptors). The rationale is that patients actively experiencing PONV may be unable to take oral medication. Also, it sometimes is necessary to block several receptor pathways responsible for PONV. If the patient continues to experience PONV, the patient and caregiver are re-informed about the possibility of narcotic-induced nausea. In the senior author's experience, most patients who fail to respond with several agents are very sensitive to narcotics and are advised to discontinue use of propoxyphene.

ANESTHESIA TECHNIQUE FOR INTRAVENOUS SEDATION

Most operations performed in the senior author's facility are performed under deep sedation using rapidly metabolized agents. The primary anesthesia medications used for deep sedation are midazolam, fentanyl, and propofol. On rare occasions small doses (25–50 mg) of ketamine (a dissociative agent) are used also. Patients are encouraged to take an oral anxiolytic (diazepam, 4–8 mg) and an oral antiemetic (aprepitant, 40 mg) with a sip of water before visiting the surgery center. Upon arrival at the facility, an initial set of vital signs is taken in the preoperative area followed by 0.1 to 0.2 mg oral clonidine (for optimization of blood pressure) with a sip of water. The dose can vary with patient medical history, body mass index, age, and scheduled procedure. If a patient presents with a systolic pressure below 90 mm Hg, the clonidine is not given.

After compression stockings are placed on the calves, the patient walks to the operating room. The patient then is placed with the head up at 45° on a Stryker eye surgery stretcher; this position minimizes initial anxiety. The stretcher allows easier access to the patient's face and neck than a conventional operating room bed. After placement and activation of the SCDs, a small (22- or 20-gauge) intravenous catheter is placed in one the antecubital veins. The rationale for placing the intravenous catheter in this site is twofold: (1) there is a lower incidence of propofol-related discomfort, and (2) intravenous catheter placement usually is less painful in this site than in the hand or other portions of the upper or lower extremities. Immediately after the intravenous catheter is inserted, a small dose of midazolam is administered (generally 2 mg intravenously; primarily for anterograde amnesia) and glycopyrolate, 0.2 mg, is administered intravenously to reduce secretions (an anticholinergic effect). The pulse oximeter is placed along with a nasal cannula running at 2 L/min, and a small dose of fentanyl (generally 25–50 μg intravenously) is given. Following this initial administration of medications, the rest of the monitors (automated blood pressure cuff, electrocardiogram monitors, electrocautery grounding pad, and end tidal CO_2 if applicable) are placed and activated. Special care is taken to make sure that the patient is adequately cushioned, the arms are properly tucked to avoid compression injuries, and the corneas are lubricated with ophthalmic ointment.

Nondiabetic patients routinely are given 6 to 10 mg dexamethasone intravenously to decrease perioperative edema and to control PONV. As the preparation of the patient continues, the propofol infusion is started, usually at 120 to 140 μg/kg/min, and is titrated downward as the case continues. When the surgeon is ready to inject the local anesthesia, a bolus of propofol is given. The oral airway then is placed with attached oxygen tubing as described earlier (see **Fig. 3**), and the oxygen is run at 2 L/min. The size of the propofol bolus ranges from 50 to 150 mg; a second dose of fentanyl (25–50 μg intravenously) may be appropriate, depending on the response to the injection.

The bulk of the case is maintained with a propofol infusion ranging from 50 to 180 μg/kg/min; one should continue to titrate the rate of infusion as the case matures. As time wears on, the dose of propofol required usually decreases because of the activity of the local anesthetic used. The key point is minimizing the total dose of propofol given while maintaining a comfortable patient. A comfortable patient is more likely to emerge smoothly and without incident. Few things are more frustrating to a surgeon than a well-executed rhytidectomy complicated by a confused, prematurely straining, bucking patient. Patients are maintained in a comfortable state of sedation until all dressings have been applied. Communication between the surgeon and the anesthesiologist or CRNA is essential for timing and smooth emergence.

Judicious administration of intravenous fluid should be used to avoid bladder distension. A typical 5-hour case requires 600 to 850 mL of intravenous fluid (lactated Ringer's solution). Also note than dexamethasone can cause diuresis and facilitate bladder filling. In prolonged surgical cases, when a full bladder is a higher probability, a urinary catheter may be required.

SUMMARY: ANESTHESIA FOR FACIAL PLASTIC SURGERY

Anesthesia for the patient undergoing facial plastic surgery can be approached in a variety of ways. This article describes a technique with which the senior author has had great success. One cannot underestimate the importance of a smooth anesthetic; this experience begins with the first preoperative phone call and continues through the recovery room stay. A patient's memories of previous bouts of PONV, awareness under anesthesia, and other perceived complications will influence the decision to undergo an elective surgical procedure.

Unfortunately, the media have sensationalized the potential for untoward events under anesthesia and have targeted elective plastic surgery in particular. When a patient expresses reluctance to undergo a procedure because of concerns about anesthesia, a consultation with the anesthesia provider often is helpful.

It is best to use the anesthetic technique with which the surgeon and anesthesia provider feel most comfortable and with which they are most experienced, but the following principles should be observed: (1) minimization of the amount of intravenous sedation or inhalation agent given; (2) adequate use of local anesthesia in the areas of dissection; (3) restriction of fluids given to avoid bladder distension; (4) aggressive management of PONV; and (5) conservative management of intraoperative hypertension. Communication between the surgeon and anesthesia personnel regarding expectations is essential. Equally important is the preoperative educational and medical preparation of the patient for the operating room.

There has been a resurgence of interest in and marketing of "facelift-type" procedures performed under local anesthesia with oral sedation. A carefully selected patient without significant aging changes can be a good physical candidate. The senior author has found, however, that many patients are not prepared psychologically to sit still in an operating room facility, aware and actively forming visual and auditory memories of a 2- to 4-h procedure. These issues should be discussed carefully with a patient before allowing the patient to commit to a procedure under local anesthesia.

The principles of patient safety and comfort are essential elements in providing anesthesia for a facial plastic surgical case. The anesthetic should be viewed as one part of the totality of care, but it is the element that inspires the most fear in patients. A well-performed anesthetic makes a smooth postoperative course more likely, but a poorly handled anesthetic can increase the likelihood of postoperative complications and can strain the relationship between surgeon and patient. There cannot be enough emphasis on making and keeping the patient happy. A happy patient will do better in the long run, will be more willing to undergo future procedures, and often provides the best form of advertisement: word of mouth.

REFERENCES

1. Donham RT. In: Eisele D, editor. Complications in head and neck surgery. 1st edition. St Louis (MO): Mosby; 1993. p. 5–25.
2. Younger D. In: Bailey B, editor. Head & neck surgery-otolaryngology. 2nd edition. Philadelphia: Lipincott-Raven; 1998. p. 147–62.
3. Camporesi EM, Greeley WJ. In: Textbook of surgery. 14th edition, Sabiston D, editor. Philadelphia: Saunders; 1991. p. 148–63.
4. Covino BG, Giddon DB. Physiology and pharmacology of local anesthetic agents. J Dent Res 1981; 60(8):1454–9.
5. Fox AJ, Rowbotham DR. Recent advances in anaesthesia. BMJ 1999;319(7209):557–60.

Volumetric Facelift with Intra- and Post-Operative Midface Volume Replacement "The Four-Dimensional Facelift"

Benjamin A. Bassichis, MD, FACS*

KEYWORDS

- Facelift • Facial fillers • Facial aging
- Midface volume restoration • Fat grafting
- Surgical technique • Cosmetic rejuvenation
- Rhytidectomy

With the millennium came an ideological shift in the approach to facial rejuvenation from predominantly subtractive surgical methods to additive volume restoration techniques.[1] Earlier facelift procedures focused on tightening lax skin, without attention to volume, often leading to a pulled post-surgical visage.[2] More recently, the effects of facial volume loss have been recognized as a central contributor to the aging process. In today's approach to facial rejuvenation, a facelift is not just a facelift but rather is a surgical make-over to restore youthful facial contour. Surgical and aesthetic studies have demonstrated the need to address the midface volume deficit when performing standard facelift techniques. Combining surgical facelift techniques with volume restoration produces a three-dimensional aesthetic improvement. In fact, nearly 95% of the author's patients undergoing facial rejuvenation surgeries receive volume correction at the time of surgery. Although the method of volume replacement can be debated and is highly operator dependant, it should be understood that this three-dimensional restoration does not adequately address the dynamic aspect of aging. The

continued treatment of the facelift patients with appropriately applied filler materials for years following surgery ensures more persistent natural results over time,[3] hence the concept of "the four-dimensional facelift." In this article, the author outlines his methodology from initial consultation, to the surgical and nonsurgical procedures, to the years of volume maintenance. The concepts of progressive treatment of facial maturation over time, of commitment, and of long-term patient care are incorporated into the author's surgical approach to the aging face to achieve enduring, natural results (Fig. 1).

UNDERSTANDING FACIAL AND MIDFACIAL AGING

During the aging process, the face loses fat and volume, and the skin loses collagen and elasticity.[4] Accentuated by full cheeks and voluptuous curves in youth, the aging face becomes framed by bony contours wrapped with thin skin, appearing deflated and aged. Understanding the dynamic facial maturation process is crucial to attaining optimal results with facial rejuvenation

Advanced Facial Plastic Surgery Center, 14755 Preston Road, Suite 110, Dallas, TX 75254, USA
* Corresponding author. Advanced Facial Plastic Surgery Center, 14755 Preston Road, Suite 110, Dallas, TX 75254.
E-mail address: drbassichis@advancedfacialplastic.com

Facial Plast Surg Clin N Am 17 (2009) 539–547
doi:10.1016/j.fsc.2009.06.004
1064-7406/09/$ – see front matter © 2009 Elsevier Inc. All rights reserved.

procedures.[1] The significant contribution of volume loss to aging features has recalibrated the manner in which the maturing face is treated. Now it is recognized that to correct the signs of facial aging, not only the skin but the facial soft tissues, the subcutaneous muscle–aponeurotic system (SMAS), fat, and even facial bones need to be addressed.

The aesthetics of the youthful face consist of healthy fullness, smooth contours, symmetry,

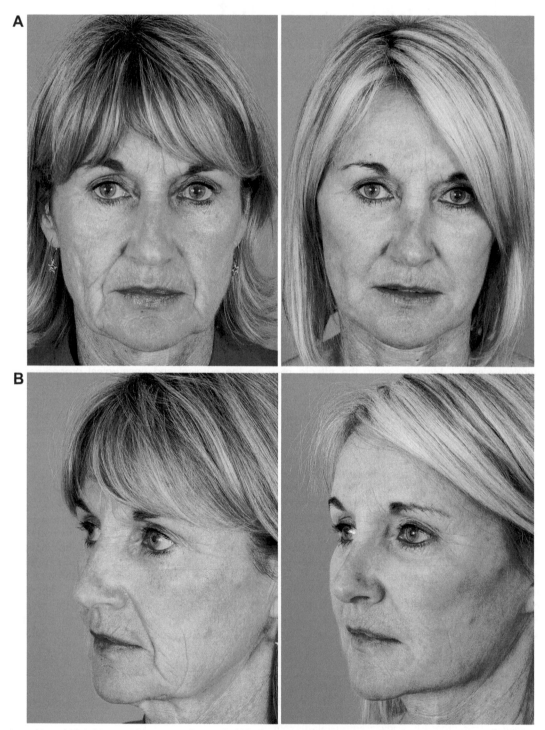

Fig. 1. (*A* and *B*) A 57-year-old woman shown (*left*) before and (*right*) 9 months after a facelift, fractionated CO2 laser resurfacing, and intraoperative filler treatments to the midface including the tear trough and mouth.

and proper proportions. The youthful midface is characterized by voluminous cheeks with an uninterrupted distribution of soft tissue overlying the malar bone and invisible transitions to neighboring facial regions. Although skin laxity yields aging effects that are most prominent along the lower face and neck, volume atrophy is most evident with midfacial aging. Here, tissue involution creates hollow infraorbital depressions and shadowing evident as dark infraorbital circles, where thinned lower eyelid skin permits visualization of the underlying blood vessels and musculature. The formerly seamless contour of soft tissue between the eyelid skin and cheek of the youthful face is interrupted by malar tissue loss with subsequent ptosis of the skin and supporting structures. Inferior migration of the malar fat pad results in a flattened, hollowed midface with pseudoherniation of lower eyelid fat pads and tear trough deformity. Concomitant atrophy of soft tissue, facial bones, and musculature evokes a skeletonized manifestation of the aging face.[5]

The modern approach to surgical rejuvenation of the face seeks to restore lost facial volume and contour to reinstate youthful facial aesthetics. Cosmetic rejuvenation of the lower face can be accomplished effectively with facelift surgery, but significantly improved aesthetic outcomes are possible when midface volume restoration is achieved and maintained over time. Even after successful facelift surgery with or without volume replacement, this loss of volume and volume shift continue to contribute significantly to the ever-progressive process of facial maturation.

MIDFACE VOLUME REPLACEMENT: A DISCUSSION OF SELECT OPTIONS

Combining facelift surgery with midface volume replacement can yield dramatic yet natural-looking improvements. The goals of midface rejuvenation in conjunction with a facelift involve reestablishing malar volume and smoothing the transition between the eyelids and cheeks. Effective restoration of volume can be difficult to accomplish in a predictable long-term manner, however. The plethora of options for midface volume restoration range from surgical techniques, including SMAS plication or midface lifts; procedures using various permutations of autologous materials, including dermis, fascia, or muscle as well as fat grafting; and alloplastic options, including malar implants, thread lifts, and injectable facial filler materials.

Surgical procedures to restore midface volume include SMAS resection, plication, or rotation;

however, these results have demonstrated minimal improvement of the naso- and mentolabial folds and negligible improvement in tear trough contour.[6] Overall, none of the myriad surgical approaches to the midface has been universally successful.

Currently, one of the more commonly used techniques for intraoperative midface volume enhancement during facelift surgery is autologous fat transfer. Although recent improvements in preparation, harvesting, and injection techniques allow longer-lasting and more predictable results,[7–10] potential issues include the need for multiple procedures, a high resorption rate, potential contour irregularities, and patient dissatisfaction. Complications that arise after fat grafting, such as lumps and bulges, overcorrection, and asymmetry, can be difficult to manage.[5] Fat grafted to the delicate tear trough and lower lid areas can be visible and palpable and can possibly worsen the contour abnormalities it was intended to correct. Used in conjunction with a facelift, fat grafting can replenish hollow cheeks, but care should be taken to avoid overcorrecting the midface, which can appear unnaturally heavy after excessive fat transfer.[11] In a slender patient who has a low body mass index, finding an adequate supply of donor fat can be a challenge, as is the increased propensity for fat reabsorpsion in these patients. In addition, weight loss or gain can alter the outcome of fat grafting. A weight loss of 10 pounds or more can result in concomitant loss of the cosmetic result achieved by the fat transfer procedure. In the reverse circumstance, the resultant fatty hypertrophy from weight gain may cause undesirable fullness or contour irregularities to the grafted material.[12] In addition, even where the static result may be successful, with facial animation such as smiling, the enhanced malar soft tissue sometimes gathers abnormally by the eye, yielding an unaesthetic appearance.

Malar implants are limited in their ability to fill the inferior orbital rim and buccal hollows and may create a relative exaggeration of these deficits. In addition, the isolated use of malar implants in an older, volume-depleted patient can accentuate a skeletonized appearance of the face.[5] Smaller implants often are preferable to replace atrophic volume loss. Medium to large implants should be reserved for the patient who desires not only to replace lost volume but also to augment a previously unsatisfactory aesthetic.[13] Overall, enthusiasm for cheek implants seems to be diminishing in favor of soft tissue–based treatments, which offer more plasticity and more natural-appearing movement than static implants.

Minimally invasive facial traction techniques, such as thread lifts, should be viewed with caution[14] because of untoward complications such as visible threads apparent through the skin surface and an often unnatural-appearing outcome.

Injectable dermal fillers are an internationally popular option for volume restoration throughout the face.[11] A broad spectrum of alloplastic injectable materials suitable for facial revolumization has been approved by the Food and Drug Administration (FDA). Because of their longevity, efficacy, safety, and reversibility, the author primarily uses hyaluronic acid (HA) products (Restylane and Restylane Perlane, Medicis Aesthetics, Scottsdale, Arizona; Juvederm Ultra and Juvederm Ultra Plus, Allergan, Irvine, California) in his practice. Other FDA-approved products, including poly-L-lactic acid (Sculptra, Dermik, Sanofi-Aventis, Bridgewater, New Jersey), collagen-based products (Cosmoderm and Cosmoplast, Allergan, Irvine, California; Evolence, ColbarLife Sciences, Herzliya, Israel), and calcium hydroxyapatite (Radiesse, BioForm Medical, San Mateo, California), provide varying degrees of longevity; however, only HA products claim reversibility through a simple injection of hyaluronidase (Amphadase, Amphastar Pharmaceuticals, Rancho Cucamonga, California; Vitrase, Ista Pharmaceuticals, Irvine, California). Also, the availability of both small- and large-particle HA products permits customization for the most effective treatments. For difficult to treat areas such as tear trough or brow, small-particle HA injections produce unsurpassed aesthetic results with experienced injection.

There are permanent injectable filler materials that can be used in an off-label capacity for correction of midface volume, such as polymethylmethacrylate (Artefill, Artes, San Diego, California) or silicone (Silikon 1000, Alcon, Fort Worth, Texas; Adaptosil 5000, Bausch Lomb, Rochester, New York). However, it should be cautioned that permanent products can yield permanent problems. Because of the need for exquisitely sensitive technique, the possibility of significant complications or corrections, and uncertain long-term risks, these permanent products are not used widely for midface revolumization, either independently or in conjunction with facelift surgery.

PREOPERATIVE EVALUATION
Initial Contact and Consultation

For every potential facelift patient, the first impression of one's practice begins during the initial telephone call or Internet inquiry. Almost independent of the quality of the surgeon's surgical skills, pleasant employees who are able to answer all patient questions effectively and knowledgeably are vital in determining whether a patient decides to establish a consultation for elective cosmetic surgery. Staff members should convey confidence and enthusiasm about their physician and medical team. Personnel with poor attitudes and an insufficient knowledge base may dissuade a potential surgical candidate.

Developing patient rapport and trust is the most important initial step in any medical consultation. To build a patient–physician relationship, the patient must feel confident in the physician's abilities and judgment. For patients, this confidence can be accomplished by openly and empathetically listening to the patient's concerns. Understanding each patient's motivation for desiring elective physical change to the face is also crucial. Patients who want to "look as young as they feel" or who are motivated to undergo surgery to enhance their own self-esteem often benefit from surgery. Patients interested in appearing refreshed to compete effectively in the job market also are successful candidates. Excluding individuals who have unrealistic expectations of surgery, those who have permutations of body dysmorphic disorders, who may be pressured to have surgery from a relative or spouse, who are unstable mentally or emotionally, or who believe that the surgery will solve a failing marriage or life problems is necessary to avoid a postoperative patient who either is unhappy or who never will be satisfied with the outcome, no matter what the result. Listening to one's own intuition regarding these red flags is as important as listening to the patient. As one of the author's respected mentors wisely stated, "You'll never regret a surgery you *didn't* do."

During a patient's initial consultation in the author's practice, the patient first has a private discussion with an aesthetic coordinator (either an aesthetician or patient coordinator) to elucidate the patient's desired aesthetic goals. The aesthetic coordinator distills the patient's information to facilitate a more productive, efficient consultation with the surgeon. In addition, the aesthetic coordinator explains the spectrum of other cosmetic services available in the practice and reviews before and after photographs with the patient to illustrate the surgeon's surgical style and to generate realistic expectations.

Armed with a synopsis of the patient's goals, the physician's facelift consultation can focus on establishing rapport and efficiently determining a treatment plan. In the author's practice, no consultation regarding full-face rejuvenation would be complete without a discussion of volume restoration. Each patient is educated regarding the necessity of long-term midface volume restoration to refresh and maintain a youthful, natural appearance. Many patients ask about longer-lasting or permanent options for volume, but, depending on body type, alloplastic products offer many advantages, most significantly reversibility and plasticity. For midface restoration in the author's practice, all FDA-approved fillers are offered in addition to fat-grafting techniques, to achieve natural full-face rejuvenation. During the patient's consultation, concepts of conservative lower eyelid fat removal and the need for long-term perpetuation of cheek volume are discussed. The author's philosophy regarding the importance of maintaining midface volume in a manner that changes dynamically as the face changes over time is central to his successful facelift outcomes. Patients understand that the midfacial volume restoration they receive at the time of facelift is not permanent, and therefore patients are not disappointed when the volume eventually dissipates. Because maintenance of volume is so crucial, the author personally performs all cosmetic injectable treatments, thereby developing strong, long-term relationships with his patients for optimal facial health.

Photographic Documentation

Digital photographs are taken of each facelift candidate including full-face frontal, left and right oblique, and right and left lateral views with attention to consistent lighting and patient positioning. Additional close-up views of the anterior neck and each ear, focusing on the pre- and post-auricular hairlines, are helpful in preoperative planning for facelift surgery. Computer image alterations are performed to illustrate potential facelift results. These images are reviewed carefully with the patient to confirm that they represent realistic, but not guaranteed, outcome scenarios.

OPERATIVE TECHNIQUE
Operative and Injection Techniques

In the operating room, the primary or revision facelift portion of the procedure of the procedure is completed. Although there are many permutations of facelift procedures, the author performs an extended sub-SMAS procedure to achieve successful lift while minimizing facial nerve concerns. This sub-SMAS technique allows some additional fullness resulting from the slight medial dog-ear in the SMAS. The mid-face portion of the SMAS is elevated with a superior vector, and the jaw line and neck region of the SMAS are repositioned posterolaterally behind the ear. After the facelift closure is sutured carefully, the facial fillers and/or fat are injected into areas requiring volume restoration. Areas to consider include cheeks/midface, nasojugal folds, tear troughs, naso- and mentolabial folds, lips, and any additional areas that are aesthetically depleted. In the midface region, one to two syringes per side of large-particle HA filler are placed deeply in the subcutaneous tissues and along the supraperiosteal plane. After injection, the HA product can be modulated manually to achieve the desired contour. Tear troughs can be rejuvenated successfully with careful injection of a small-particle HA filler placed just beneath the dermis. When treating superficial and delicate areas such as the tear trough, conservative dermal product placement is crucial, because superficial injection can be visible through the skin, worsening the patient's appearance.[1] In the lower face, including the naso- and mentolabial folds, two to three syringes of small-particle filler are injected as cosmetically indicated (**Fig. 2** A and B).

Two factors paramount to successful filler injections are treating to complete correction and filler placement in the dermis. Except for the periorbital and tear trough areas, where prudent undercorrection is the rule, both the patient and the surgeon are more likely to be satisfied with the treatment outcomes when complete correction is achieved. Anecdotally, experienced injectors have recognized that if complete correction is accomplished initially, the correction persists longer.[1] After completing the filler injections, standard post-facelift pressure dressings are applied using fluffs, Kerlex rolls, and Coban dressings.

Maintenance of Results

During the initial consultation for full-face rejuvenation, patients are educated regarding the need for continued volume replacement to maintain results. To optimize the longevity of the filler injections, the initial re-treatment should be performed between 4.5 and 9 months after surgery.[15] Additional follow-up treatments are scheduled yearly or as needed to maintain the most ideal, customized result.

DISCUSSION: FACELIFT WITH MIDFACE VOLUME

Although previous facelift techniques focused on tightening loose skin and resuspending descended structures, most of these techniques did not address the loss of midfacial volume. For some patients, loss of youthful facial fullness can be the most significant sign of aging. In approaching full-face rejuvenation effectively, a combination of traction and volume can achieve the most natural-appearing results.

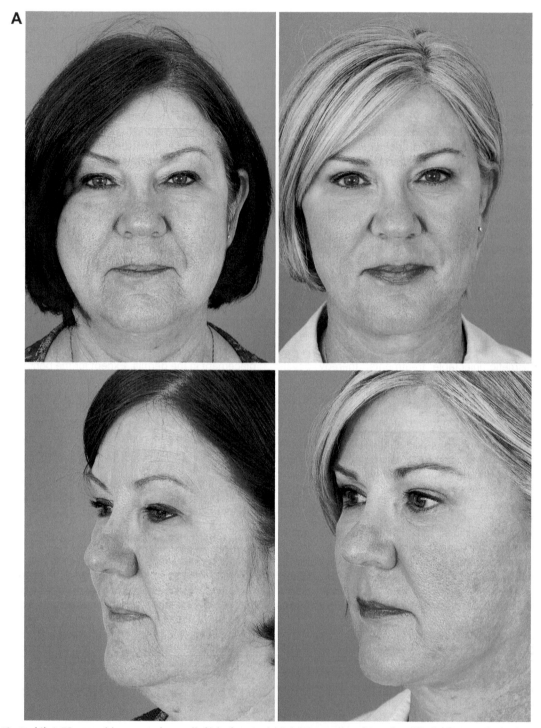

Fig. 2. (*A*) A 52-year-old woman shown (*left*) before and (*right*) 9 months after a facelift, fractionated CO2 laser resurfacing, and intraoperative filler treatments to the midface, including the tear trough, lips, and nasolabial folds. (*B*) A 46-year-old woman shown before and 12 months after a facelift, browlift, upper and lower blepharoplasty, and intraoperative filler treatments to the midface including the tear trough and nasolabial and perioral areas.

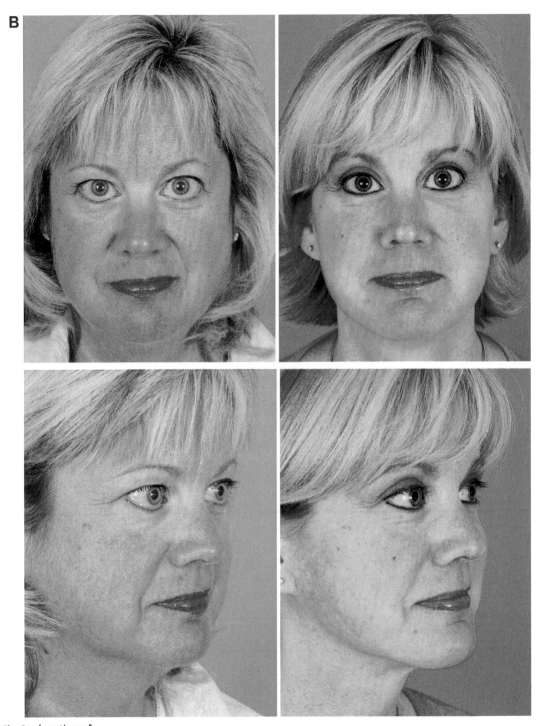

Fig. 2. (*continued*)

Natural-looking and dynamic restoration of volume can be a challenging prospect. The unrelenting atrophy of facial volume occurs at multiple levels, in various tissue types, and with variable velocities. As such, there currently is no single, one-time technology to address this changing system effectively in a fully predictable fashion. Injectable facial fillers provide the natural-appearing volume to address facial atrophy and use the potential downside of impermanence to an advantage, permitting customized, adaptive results. Studies also have shown that injected HA fillers can stimulate dermal fibroblasts to produce collagen,

yielding potential long-term volume results over time.[16]

Although numerous variations of facelift techniques are possible, the author has chosen to

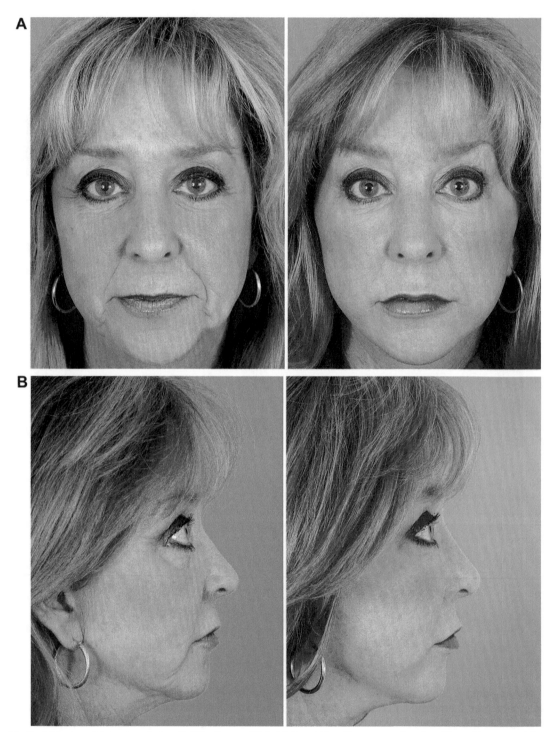

Fig. 3. A 62-year-old woman shown (*left*) before and (*right*) 5 months after a secondary facelift and intraoperative HA filler treatments to the midface including the tear trough, nasolabial and perioral areas (*A, B*).

focus this article on the vital concept of combined facelift plus midface volume restoration rather than a debate about facelift surgical technique. In the earlier phase of his practice, when volume played a small role during surgical procedures, to the present, when 95% of full-face rejuvenation procedures receive concomitant volume replacement, the author has noted a definite evolution in facelift paradigm culminating in this combined approach. This described technique has shown significant volumetric improvement and offers less risk for complications, especially those involving facial nerves. The simultaneous addition of volume sometimes is even more significant at the time of revision surgery or secondary facelifts, because additional contour abnormalities may require correction during these procedures (**Fig. 3**).

In addition, the temporal component of this method addresses the dynamic nature of facial maturation and allows a healthy, long-term commitment to facial rejuvenation. Albert Einstein theorized that time was the fourth dimension[17]; hence, the concept of integrating time into a three-dimensional facial restoration yields the "four-dimensional facelift."

Although the search for the perfect long-lasting and dynamic midfacial rejuvenation continues, the present understanding of facial aging and the current state of technology make the approach described herein a contemporary and effective option for full-face rejuvenation.

SUMMARY

The twenty-first century approach to the surgical treatment of facial aging is customized to match each patient's aesthetic needs and desires. The significant contribution of volume loss to aging features has recalibrated the manner in which the maturing face is treated. Modern facial plastic surgery has come a long way from the more limited traction-centered approach, to achieve dynamic, volumetric, natural-looking outcomes that are truly rejuvenating. Viewed as a "four-dimensional" process, the continued treatment of facelift patients with appropriately applied filler materials for years after the surgical procedure can achieve more persistent, natural-looking outcomes.

ACKNOWLEDGMENTS

This manuscript is dedicated to Dr William Bassichis and Dr Joseph Mantel. Thank you to Dr Michelle Mantel Bassichis for her assistance with this project.

REFERENCES

1. Dayan SH, Bassichis BA. Facial dermal fillers: selection of appropriate products and techniques. Aesthet Surg J 2008;28(3):335–47.
2. Ellenbogen R, Youn A, Yamini D, et al. The volumetric facelift. Aesthet Surg J 2004;24:514–22.
3. Panfilov DE, editor. Introduction: aesthetic surgery of the facial mosaic. Heidelberg: Springer-Verlag; 2007. p. 3–4.
4. Gilchrest BA. Cellular and molecular changes in aging skin. J Geriatr Dermatol 1994;2:3–6.
5. DeFatta RJ, Williams EF. Fat transfer in conjunction with facial rejuvenation procedures. Facial Plast Surg Clin North Am 2008;16(4):383–90.
6. Coleman SR. Structural fat grafts: the ideal filler? Clin Plast Surg 2001;28(1):111–9.
7. Coleman SR. Facial reconstruction with lipostructure. Clin Plast Surg 1997;24:347–67.
8. Amar RE. Microinfiltration of the fat cells of the face or reconstruction of the tissue with grafts of fat tissue. Ann Chir Plast Esthet 1999;44: 593–608.
9. Guerrerosantos J, Gonzalez–Mendoza A, Masmela Y, et al. Long term survival of free fat grafts in muscle: an experimental study in rats. Aesthetic Plast Surg 1996; 20:403–8.
10. Rohrich RJ, Sorokin ES, Brown SA. In search of improved fat transfer viability; a quantitative analysis of the role of centrifugation and harvest site. Plast Reconstr Surg 2004;113:391–5.
11. Lambros V. Models of facial aging and implications for treatment. Clin Plast Surg 2008;35(3):319–27.
12. Obagi S. Autologous fat augmentation: a perfect fit in new and emerging technologies. Facial Plast Surg Clin North Am 2007;15(2):221–8.
13. Chisholm BB. Facial implants: facial augmentation and volume restoration. Facial Plast Surg Clin North Am 2008;16(4):467–74.
14. Downs BW, Wang TD. Current concepts in midfacial rejuvenation. Curr Opin Otolaryngol Head Neck Surg 2008;16(4):335–8.
15. Narins RS, Dayan SH, Brandt FS, et al. Persistence and improvement of nasolabial fold correction with nonanimal-stabilized hyaluronic acid 100,000 gel particles/mL filler on two retreatment schedules: results up to 18 months on two retreatment schedules. Dermatol Surg 2008;34:S2–8.
16. Wang F, Garza LA, Kang S, et al. In vivo stimulation of denovo collagen production caused by cross-linked hyaluronic acid dermal filler injections in photodamaged human skin. Arch Dermatol 2007;143(2):155–63.
17. Einstein A, Beck A. The collected papers of Albert Einstein. Princeton (NJ): Princeton University Press; 1987.

Short-Scar Purse-String Facelift

Amir M. Karam, MD[a,b,*], L. Mike Nayak, MD[c,d],
Samuel M. Lam, MD[e]

KEYWORDS

- Facial rejuvenation • Facelift • Purse-string facelift
- MACS lift • S-lift • Neck lift • SMAS facelift

Despite the variety of novel and sophisticated facial rejuvenation technologies available today, management of the lower face and neck remains primarily surgical in nature. The reference standard treatment for correction of the senescent jaw line and neck is a rhytidectomy.

The evolution of modern facelift surgery has followed an interesting and dynamic course with many milestones and factors that have influenced current thinking about the ideal facelift operation. In many ways, the course has come full circle from the original skin-only rhytidectomy approaches of the early 1900s, through the more complex sub- subcutaneous muscle–aponeurotic system (SMAS) techniques used from the late 1970s through most of the 1990s.[1–6] The paradigm began to shift slowly as surgeons began to realize that bigger operations do not necessarily result in better results. In fact, in face of the higher complication rates and morbidity, several surgeons began to question the utility and rationale for the conventional facelift techniques involving deep-plane or sub-SMAS dissections.

In the late 1990s, Daniel Baker and Zia Saylan popularized the lateral SMASectomy and the S-lift, respectively.[7,8] Both these techniques incorporate a short incision approach coupled with a supra-SMAS dissection plane and a largely vertically oriented vector of SMAS elevation. These novel techniques illustrated the potential for excellent, naturally enhancing results, decreased potential morbidity, and surgical expediency.

PURSE-STRING FACELIFT

Saylan's S-lift was the first purse-string facelift and involved an SMAS plication technique that was intended to provide an even less invasive facelift procedure. It featured a short, preauricular-only incision, short flap, and double purse-string sutures that were anchored to the periosteum of the posterolateral zygomatic arch. The procedure was intended to be performed under local anesthesia, a consideration that was appealing to many patients. Although the technique was considerably more conservative, it delivered efficacious results for both men and women between the ages of 40 and 50 years. The most obvious shortcoming was the inability to improve significantly the cervicomental angle and overall neck laxity.

Tonnard and Verpaele's minimal access cranial suspension (MACS) lift, described in 2001, was a significant advance in purse-sting facelift technique. By performing additional undermining onto the lateral face and jowl region, adding judicious submental liposuction, and using larger purse-sting sutures to capture the cranial border of the platysma more effectively, overall results were improved, especially in heavier faces and those

[a] Carmel Valley Facial Plastic Surgery, 4765 Carmel Mountain Road, Suite 201, San Diego, CA 92130, USA
[b] Division of Otolaryngology-Head and Neck Surgery, Department of Surgery, University of California, 350 Dickinson Street, Suite 211, San Diego, CA 92130, USA
[c] Nayak Plastic Surgery and Skin Enhancement Center, 763 S. New Ballas Road, Suite 204, St Louis, MO 63141, USA
[d] Department of Otolaryngology-Head and Neck Surgery, St Louis University, St Louis, MO, USA
[e] Willow Bend Wellness Center & Lam Facial Plastics, 6101 Chapel Hill Boulevard, Suite 101, Plano, TX 75093, USA
* Corresponding author.
E-mail address: md@drkaram.com (A.M. Karam).

Facial Plast Surg Clin N Am 17 (2009) 549–556
doi:10.1016/j.fsc.2009.06.007

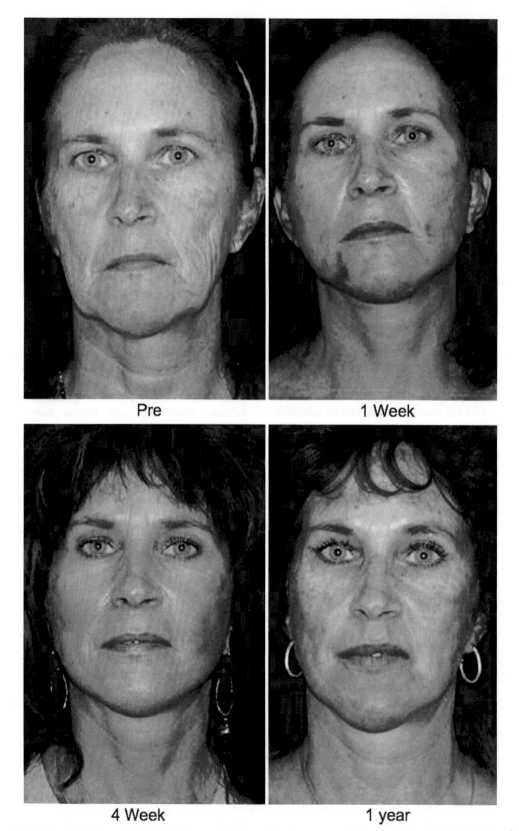

Pre   1 Week

4 Week   1 year

Fig. 1. A series of photographs taken before and after a short-scar purse-string facelift and limited submento-plasty. Note the limited edema and minimal ecchymosis 1 week postoperatively. Despite the significant degree of photodamage and loss of skin elasticity, the results remain durable over the 1-year period. (*Photographs cour-tesy of* L. Mike Nayak, MD, St Louis, MO.)

with more cervicomental laxity than the S-lift could correct.

In June 2004, Brandy introduced a modification of Saylan's S-lift.[9,10] Since then, the operation has continued to be refined. Compared with the original S-lift, Brandy's modified purse-string facelift involves postauricular undermining and undermining of a larger region in the lateral neck, more aggressively correcting the platysma-SMAS complex. The lift is more vertically oriented than the S-lift, further correcting the cervical laxity. The ability to correct greater degrees of neck and jowl laxity broadens the indications to include individuals of all ages. The authors' work is based largely on this modification, and they owe credit to Brandy for the advances he has made in the purse-string facelift.

The purse strings themselves also are different from those used in the S-lift or MACS lift; in this case, they are concentric, with a smaller, central purse string pretightening the face and drawing even more of the cranial edge of the platysma into the field to be captured definitively by the larger, eccentric, second purse-string suture. This double encircling purse-string suture allows

progressive, incremental tightening and also creates a favorable fullness at the region of the gonial angle, which often is deficient in aging faces.

To date, the results have been extremely gratifying (**Figs. 1–3**), with very high patient satisfaction. Naturally, the durability of the results always must be questioned when evaluating a novel technique. Although the 1-year photographs shown here illustrate the anatomic stability of the surgical outcomes, several studies have evaluated this concept in comparative studies. In 1996, Aston and colleagues[11] performed a prospective comparison of limited incision and limited dissection techniques (lateral SMASectomy and standard SMAS) versus more extensive techniques (composite and extended SMAS facelifts). The results did not show a detectable difference in outcomes between these techniques. The investigators concluded that the increased morbidity, surgical risks, and convalescence associated with these more extensive approaches may not be warranted in the average facelift patient. Later, Prado and colleagues[12] published a split-face study comparing the lateral SMASectomy with the MACS lift (purse-string facelift). In this study,

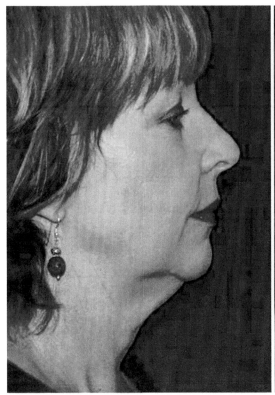
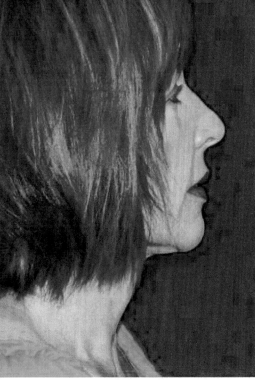

Before   1 year post

Fig. 2. Photographs taken before and 1 year after a short-scar purse-string facelift and limited submentoplasty. (*Photographs courtesy of* L. Mike Nayak, MD, St Louis, MO.)

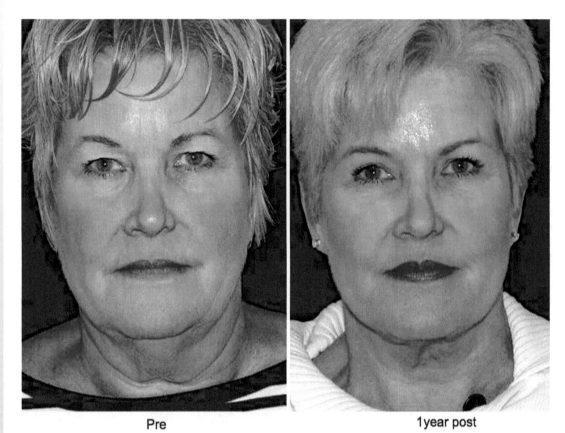

Pre   1year post

Fig. 3. Photographs taken before and 1 year after a short-scar purse-string facelift, limited submentoplasty, and four-lid blepharoplasty. (*Photographs courtesy of* L. Mike Nayak, MD, St Louis, MO.)

there was no detectable difference in result durability at 2 years between the SMASectomy and the purse string facelift side. The overall conclusion of these studies is that, as long as the SMAS and platysma are fundamentally repositioned and stabilized, the results will be meaningful and enduring. As an extension of this concept, the choice of technique should be based on achieving the best results with the least risk, morbidity, and convalescence.

SURGICAL TECHNIQUE
Surgical Markings

Fig. 4A illustrates the typical incision marking used, beginning with a short, intensively beveled preauricular trichophytic incision that continues into a preauricular, post-tragal incision. This incision then continues for a variable degree into a postauricular incision. In patients who have mild laxity or excellent skin tone, the incision may terminate at the base of the conchal bowl. In very lax, photodamaged skin, the incision probably will need to be carried up to the helix-hair touch-point and then back down the hairline as

a beveled, trichophytic occipital hair-edge incision. Average undermining distances then are drawn 5 cm anterior to the tragus incision line, 5.5 cm anterior to the earlobe along the angle of the mandible, and 6 cm inferior to the earlobe. In general, the less elastic the skin, the more prone it is to postoperative "sweeping" from a strictly vertical lift, and the more aggressive the skin undermining must be to prevent this outcome (**Fig. 4**B).

OPERATIVE TECHNIQUE
Anesthesia

When the procedure is performed under local anesthesia, diazepam (10 mg) is administered orally, and a combination of midazolam (2.5 mg) and meperidine hydrochloride (50 mg) is given intramuscularly before the initiation of the procedure.

The patient then is brought into the operating room, and the face is prepped with povidone-iodine solution. The area to be undermined is infiltrated with 0.25% lidocaine hydrochloride with 1:400,000 epinephrine using a 21-gauge spinal

A

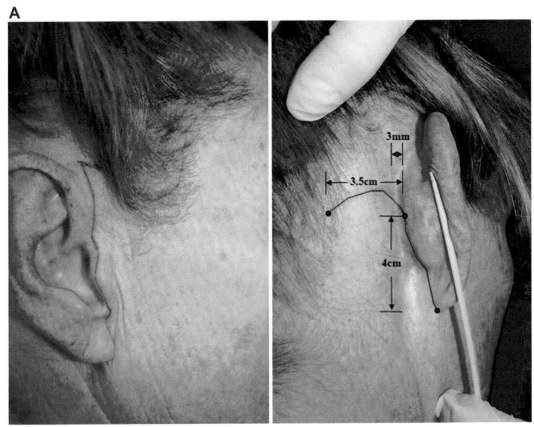

Fig. 4. (*A*) Surgical markings are begun on the tragus and extend along the front of the ear and 3 mm behind the temporal hairline. Notice how the line meanders along the anatomy of the ear, creating a much less detectable scar. The line is extended 2 mm above the posterior earlobe crease and is 4 cm in length. The hockey stick usually is 1.5 cm to 3.5 cm in length but varies in size depending on the amount of excessive posterior neck skin available for Burrow's triangle excision during the procedure. (*B*) Outline of the extent of subcutaneous undermining. The undermining should be 1 cm below the inferior border of the brow, 5 cm anterior to the tragus parallel to the floor, 5.5 cm anterior to the earlobe along the mandible, 6 cm directly inferior to the earlobe, and 2.5 to 4.0 cm away from the earlobe crease. (*Courtesy of* Dominic Brandy, MD, Pittsburgh, PA.)

needle and making certain to remain in the subcutaneous space.

At this point, in patients who have superficial submental fat, a standard submental liposuction is preformed. In patients who have a moderate degree of submental platysmal banding, a medial platysmaplasty is preformed to the level of the hyoid after the elevation of a submental skin flap. Back cuts are made in the platysma to enhance the cervicomental angle.

Next, an incision is initiated at the temporal hairline. Subcutaneous undermining is begun with a Bard-Parker No.15 blade and then is completed using the facelift scissors. The most critical aspect of the skin undermining is to make certain that the flap is not excessively thin at the predicted site where the V-shaped advanced flap opposes the scalp (at the superior attachment of the pinna). This region is most susceptible to necrosis and

should be as thick as possible, without capturing the superficial temporoparietal fascia. When all the undermining is completed, thorough hemostasis is accomplished.

At this point in the procedure, the encircling double purse-string SMAS plication is performed. First, 0.25% lidocaine hydrochloride with 1:400,000 epinephrine is injected into the site of the anchor sutures. These injections are performed with a 1-inch 30-gauge needle and are extended all the way down to the zygomatic arch 1.5 cm away from the skin edge of the tragus, a course that should be safely behind the expected course of the frontal branch of the facial nerve. The choice of suture depends on the surgeon's performance and ranges from 2–0 green braided nylon (EthiBond, Ethicon Inc, Somerville, NJ) to 0 or 1 purple polydioxanone. The anchoring suture is placed 1.5 cm away from the skin edge,

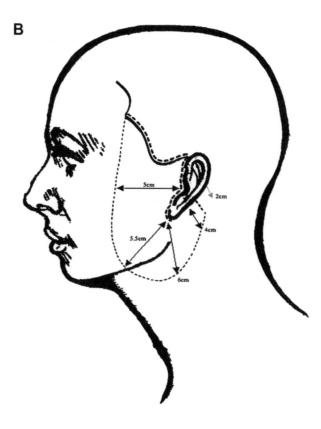

B

Fig. 4. (*continued*)

directly over the posterior zygomatic arch (**Fig. 5**). The suture needle should scrape bone and should grasp the periosteum before surfacing. The posterosuperior position of the first purse string is the anchor stitch. The diameter of this purse string is about 4 to 5 cm, and it extends down to the cranial portion of the platysma (just below the angle of the mandible). Each bite is roughly 1.5 cm long and should be deep enough to engage the fibrous

SMAS (not just subcutaneous fat) but not so deep as to jeopardize the facial nerve.

The second anchoring stitch is performed eccentric to the first. The needle enters 3 mm above and 3 mm medial to the knot of the first purse string. This anchor suture is placed in the periosteum of the zygomatic arch similar to the first suture. Four to five 1.5-cm-long grasps through the SMAS are taken in a directly inferior

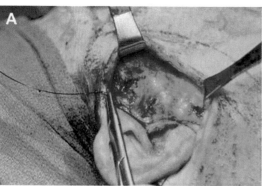
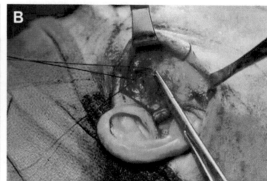

Fig. 5. Intraoperative view. The newer encircling double purse-string plication technique involves first performing an anchor suture 1.5 cm away from the skin edge. This anchor suture is directly over the zygomatic arch, passes all the way to the bone, and is 1.5 cm in length (*A*, *B*).

direction (**Fig. 6**B), taking care to continue well beyond the angle of the mandible before turning anteriorly to ensure the capture of several solid bites of the cranial border of the platysma in the submandibular region. The remainder of the 1.5-cm-long grasps follows the outer edge of the undermined zone toward the periorbital region (**Fig. 6**B). The first four grasps along the line of undermining tighten platysma; the remaining grasps tighten the SMAS. Note the overlapping of the grasps in the lower neck and midface areas (**Fig. 6**A and B). These overlaps prevent rip-through in an area where the tissues sometimes can be frail.

When the second purse string arrives at the height as its origin anchor suture, 1.5-cm grasps of SMAS are made toward this higher anchor suture (3 mm above the first anchor suture). The last grasp, before meeting the second anchor suture, should be a third anchor suture creating a V-shaped double anchoring point for the larger second purse-string suture. This third anchor suture is not as deep as the first two but should at least be 3 mm deep. Once again, five throws of the suture are made, and a 2-mm suture end is left.

As soon as the encircling double purse string is completed, thorough hemostasis is accomplished, and the redundant skin is excised. The skin drape vector can vary from patient to patient. Although the vector usually has a predominantly vertical direction, in patients who have extensive photoaging, a more posterior skin drape may be required to prevent upward striae in the healing skin flap. The flap is inset using a combination of deep 5–0 polydioxanone sutures. The deep sutures from the temporal hairline to the superior attachment of the ear are tacked down to the

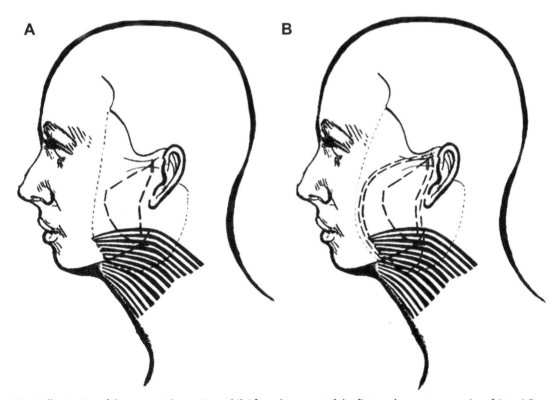

Fig. 6. Illustration of the purse-string pattern. (*A*) After placement of the first anchor suture, a series of 1- to 1.5-cm bites of fibrous SMAS starts posteriorly and extends down toward the angle of the mandible and then back up toward the anchor point. The diameter of this first purse string is 4 to 5 cm. (*B*) The second 1.5-cm anchor suture (indicated by the heavy dashed lines in the upper preauricular region) starts 3 mm superior and 3 mm lateral to the knot of the first anchor suture's knot. Four to five 1.5-cm-long grasps of SMAS are made in a directly inferior direction. The next four 1.5-cm-long grasps will be of platysma and should follow directly behind the edge of skin undermining. Once the surgeon has reached the same height as the superior aspect of the second anchor suture, superficial grasps are made directly toward the second anchor suture. The last grasp of tissue before hitting the second anchor suture will be the third anchor suture and should be 3 mm deep. The second and third anchor sutures thus will create a V-shaped anchoring point for the platysma, jowl, and midface. (*Courtesy of* Dominic Brandy, MD, Pittsburgh, PA.)

temporalis fascia. These tacking sutures are critical for stabilization and anchoring of the flap. Once these sutures are completed, the 5–0 polydioxanone sutures are placed throughout the length of the remaining incision. After all deep sutures are placed, the skin is sutured with a running 6–0 fast-absorbing gut suture.

Patients are asked to wash the incisions three times per day with a mild soap. Antibiotic ointment is applied to all incisions for 4 to 5 days. Antibiotics typically are prescribed. A cold compress is placed under the chin strap for the first 2 to 3 days. At 1 week, the patient can apply water-based makeup to all incision sites. Patients are seen 1 week, 6 weeks, 3 months, and 1 year postoperatively.

COMPLICATIONS

Complications were found to be rare with this approach. The authors experienced a 1% incidence of flap skin necrosis (>1 cm^2) at the level of the superior helix. Conservative wound care was used with spontaneous resolution. Hematomas requiring evacuation occurred at a rate of 1% and were managed by simple aspiration in the office on postoperative day 1 without the need for re-exploration. Hypertrophic scarring of the postauricular incision occurred in 1% of the cases and was managed with steroid injection without complication or need for scar revision. There were no cases of permanent or temporary facial nerve weakness. All patients had temporary anesthesia over the undermined area that resolved in approximately 3 months.

SUMMARY

A variety of surgical approaches exist for rejuvenating the lower face and neck. When comparing these approaches, it is tempting to focus primarily on the potential results each of these procedures can achieve. It is equally, if not more important, however, to remember that these procedures are elective and cosmetic, and it is essential to balance the risk–benefit ratio when comparing operative techniques. Patients today are less accepting of long downtimes and relatively high-risk exposure; they want meaningful results achieved in the safest way possible. In the authors' experience, many patients prefer improvement over perceived perfection, if the former involves less downtime, less risk, and a lower potential of an unnatural or overoperated appearance. Because of its vertical advancement, the vertical purse-string facelift combines the simplicity and safety of a superficial rhytidectomy while providing substantial rejuvenating outcomes to the lower face, neck, and midface. Similar to Tonnard's MACS-Lift and Baker's lateral SMASectomy, the vertical vector used in this procedure produces significant rejuvenative results. Use of the deep fascia overlying the lateral periosteum as an anchor point provides a stable fixation point for the double purse-string plication sutures. Patient recovery ranges from 1 to 2 weeks. The potential for serious long-term complication (ie, motor nerve damage or distorted facial soft tissue contour) is limited. To date, consistency and patient satisfaction have been extremely high.

REFERENCES

1. Lexer E. Zur Gesichtplastik [comment]. Arch Klin Chir 1910;92:749.
2. Joseph J. Plastic operation on the protruding cheek [comment]. Dtch Med Wochenschr 1921;47:287.
3. Ramirez OM, Pozner JM. Subperiosteal minimally invasive laser endoscopic rhytidectomy: the SMILE facelift. Aesthetic Plast Surg 1996;20(6):463–70.
4. Toledo LS. Video-endoscopic facelift. Aesth Plast Surg 1994;18(2):149–52.
5. Hamra ST. Composite rhytidectomy. Plast Reconstr Surg 1992;90:1–13.
6. Ullmann Y, Levy Y. Superextended facelift: our experience with 3,580 patients. Ann Plast Surg 2004; 52(1):8–14.
7. Baker DC. Lateral SMASectomy. Plast Reconstr Surg 1997;100:509–13.
8. Saylan Z. The S-lift for facial rejuvenation. Int J Cosm Surg 1999;7(1):18–23.
9. Brandy DA. The QuickLift: a modification of the s-lift. Cosmet Dermatol 2004;17:251–360.
10. Brandy DA. The Quicklift™: featuring an encircling double purse-string plication technique with blunt neck/jowl undermining for tightening of the sagging SMAS, platysma and skin. Am J Cosmet Surg 2005; 22(4):223–32.
11. Ivy EJ, Lorenc ZP, Aston SJ. Is there a difference? A prospective study comparing lateral and standard SMAS face lifts with extended SMAS and composite rhytidectomies. Plast Reconstr Surg 1996;98(7): 1135–43 [discussion: 1144–7].
12. Prado A, Andrades P, Danilla S, et al. A clinical retrospective study comparing two short-scar face lifts: minimal access cranial suspension versus lateral SMASectomy. Plast Reconstr Surg 2006;117(5): 1413–25 [discussion: 1426–7].

Deep Plane Rhytidectomy and Variations

Shan R. Baker, MD[a,b,*]

KEYWORDS

- Deep plane facelift • Mid-facelift • SUB-SMAS facelift
- SMAS lift • Facelift • Subperiosteal facelift

It was not until the 1970s that significant innovations in facelifting were introduced. This was initiated by the work of Skoog who reported dissecting beneath the superficial fascia of the face.[1] Before 1974, rhytidectomy had consisted of a simple subcutaneous dissection of facial and cervical skin with or without suture suspension of the underlying superficial fascia. Skoog[2] demonstrated that an advancement flap dissected beneath the superficial fascia, later to be named the "superficial musculoaponeurotic system" (SMAS), while leaving the overlying skin attached, could improve the jaw line better than a subcutaneous dissection of the skin. Skoog's discovery that enhanced results were possible from dissecting deeper than the conventional subcutaneous tissue plane ushered in a renaissance for rhytidectomy, and today surgeons are in the midst of this renaissance. A variety of dissection planes deeper than the conventional subcutaneous tissue plane are discussed in this article.

The SMAS is essentially a fascial extension of the platysmal muscle beneath the cheek fat of the midface.[3–5] Traction placed on the SMAS is not transmitted to the melolabial fold and as a consequence does not ameliorate the fold. This is because the SMAS is effectively anchored by the bony origins of the mimetic muscles it envelops. Recent evidence suggests that the SMAS dissipates before reaching the zygomatic major muscle.[6] This knowledge does not alter the requirement to release the investments of the SMAS in the region of the midface to move the SMAS and the overlying cheek fat upward, however, thereby improving the melolabial fold and the appearance of the midface.[7] The deep plane rhytidectomy perfected by Hamra[8] extended a sub-SMAS dissection of the inferior cheek superiorly, cutting through the SMAS peripherally, and releasing it from its superomedial investments of the midface so that the SMAS and the overlying skin and subcutaneous tissues could be advanced upward as a single tissue flap. Release of the SMAS was accomplished by transitioning from a sub-SMAS plane in the inferior cheek to a supra-SMAS plane in the superior medial cheek remaining just superficial to the zygomatic major and minor muscles (**Fig. 1**).[9] The dissection extended medially beyond the melolabial fold, totally releasing all SMAS attachments to the dermis of the upper lip and creating a thick musculocutaneous flap composed of skin, subcutaneous fat of the cheek, and the platysma. Hamra[10] subsequently modified the deep plane rhytidectomy by including the orbicularis occuli in the rhytidectomy flap and termed it a "composite rhytidectomy." Owsley[11] showed that by dissecting medially from the malar eminence to the lateral upper lip just superficial to the SMAS in the plane immediately above the orbicularis occuli, zygomaticus, and levator muscles, the cheek fat could be suspended superiorly, restoring a youthful appearance to the midface

[a] Section of Facial Plastic and Reconstructive Surgery, Department of Otolaryngology-Head and Neck Surgery, University of Michigan, 1500 East Medical Center Drive, 1904 Taubman Center, Ann Arbor, MI 48109–5312, USA
[b] University of Michigan, Center for Facial Cosmetic Surgery, 19900 Haggerty Road, Suite 103, Livonia, MI 48152, USA
* University of Michigan, Center for Facial Cosmetic Surgery, 19900 Haggerty Road, Suite 103, Livonia, MI 48152.
E-mail address: shanb@med.umich.edu

Facial Plast Surg Clin N Am 17 (2009) 557–573
doi:10.1016/j.fsc.2009.06.003
1064-7406/09/$ – see front matter © 2009 Elsevier Inc. All rights reserved.

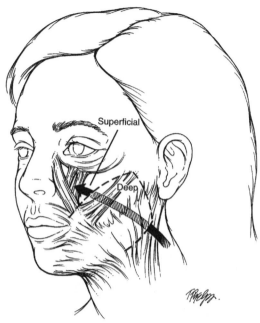

Fig. 1. The deep plane rhytidectomy described by Hamra[8] extended a sub-SMAS dissection of the inferior cheek superiorly, cutting through the SMAS peripherally, releasing the SMAS from investments to the midface muscles so that the SMAS and overlying skin and cheek fat could be mobilized upward. This release was accompanied by transitioning from a deep (sub-SMAS) plane in the inferior cheek to a superficial (supra-SMAS) plane in the superior medial cheek. (*From* Baker SR. Rhytidectomy. In: Cummings CW, Flint PW, Harker LA, et al, editors. Otolaryngology-head and neck surgery, vol. 1. Philadelphia: Elsevier; 2008.)

and effacing the melolabial fold. He showed that a sub-SMAS dissection was not at all necessary to improve the midface. Owsley's approach is often referred to as an "extended supra-SMAS rhytidectomy."

Advancement of the cheek fat superolaterally is necessary to improve the midface, whereas a sub-SMAS dissection with mobilization of a composite flap of platysma and overlying skin is beneficial for correcting the jowl. Dissection beneath the SMAS of the inferior cheek is readily accomplished with blunt dissection once the SMAS has been incised. Shifting the dissection to a more superficial plane as one extends superiorly from beneath the platysma of the lower cheek to a plane superficial to the SMAS in the midface is tedious, however, and must be performed sharply. By necessity, the surgeon must make a transition from one surgical plane to another and risk injury to the zygomatic branch of the facial nerve. In addition, to mobilize the ptotic cheek fat upward in the midface, a lengthy anterior dissection over the convexity

of the zygoma is necessary. The convexity often prevents direct visualization of the dissection.

The knowledge gained from the clinical and anatomic studies performed in the mid and late 1970s enabled continued refinement of sub-SMAS and extended supra-SMAS dissection techniques, culminating in the early 1990s. Emerging in parallel with these surgical approaches was the development of a different concept for rejuvenating the midface accomplished by a subperiosteal dissection. In 1980, Tessier[12] demonstrated that undermining the periosteum of the superior and lateral orbital rim allowed elevation of the soft tissues of the forehead and eyebrows, with improved results compared with previous techniques for forehead lifting. In 1988, Psillakis and colleagues[13] reported on a subperiosteal rhytidectomy technique that involved detachment of all periosteum from the bony orbital rims, upper maxilla, zygoma, and nose. Following this detachment the soft tissues of the forehead, lateral canthus, midface including the melolabial folds, and to some degree the jowls, were lifted to re-establish a more youthful relationship with the underlying facial skeleton. Because of troubling temporary forehead paralysis from trauma to the temporal branch of the facial nerve (6.7%), the authors advocated restricting subperiosteal dissection of the zygomatic arch to the anterior third to reduce the risk of injury. Ramirez and colleagues[14] modified the subperiosteal facelift described by Psillakis and colleagues[13] permitting significant improvement in the safety and clinical results. They released the periosteum from the entire zygomatic arch by dissecting deep to the temporalis fascia. The temporalis fascia was then used as a lifting and anchoring element of the entire cheek and perioral soft tissues. The surgical approach by Ramirez and colleagues[14] showed improved midface suspension by complete subperiosteal undermining of the midfacial bones. The suspension seemed to have the same influence on the melolabial fold as the deep plane facelift; specifically, elevation of the ptotic cheek fat to a more youthful position with effacement of the fold.

The subperiosteal approach had the advantage of rejuvenating the midface without placing unnatural tension on the skin in the temporal area. This tension is necessary when using an extended supra-SMAS or deep plane rhytidectomy to pull the cheek fat with the overlying skin upward. In contrast, the subperiosteal approach placed traction on the periosteum to maintain repositioning of the midface tissues. It also did not require a long cheek flap extending anteriorly beyond the convexity of the zygoma as called for by the deep plane and extended supra-SMAS facelifts. The extensive release of the periosteum away from the zygoma and maxilla allowed better elevation of the upper lip and corner of the mouth by moving the origin of the zygomatic musculature to a higher position on the zygoma. This effectively "shortens" the zygomatic musculature, which lifts the oral commissure upward, producing a more pleasant shape to the mouth. This maneuver cannot be accomplished with sub-SMAS or extended supra-SMAS dissections. Finally, in individuals with early facial aging, the subperiosteal approach through endoscopic techniques offered a method of lifting the face without skin excisions and the resulting preauricular scar.

The subperiosteal facelift described by Ramirez and colleagues[14] is technically difficult because it requires a temporal approach, which is considerably removed from the body of the zygoma and the anterior maxilla where the midface soft tissues are attached. As with the deep plane rhytidectomy, visibility anterior to the convexity of the zygoma is limited and it may be necessary to perform some dissection blindly. Because the temporal approach by itself presented difficulties with detachment of the periosteum from the maxilla, surgeons turned to other approaches. The most popular of these was transorbital access to the midface achieved by performing a lower lid blepharoplasty using a transcutaneous or transconjunctival approach. Through the blepharoplasty incision, the periosteum was released from the maxilla and zygoma and the soft tissues of the midface suspended either to a periosteal cuff at the inferior bony orbital rim or to the temporalis fascia in the anteroinferior aspect of the temporal fossa.[15–18] A major drawback of the transorbital route was not infrequent problems of lower lid retraction or even ectropion. This complication occurs from trauma to the orbicularis occuli and subsequent scar contracture. To reduce this risk some surgeons recommended concomitant lateral canthoplasty, or at the very least canthopexy. Other surgeons avoided this risk all together by combining a transtemporal and transoral approach and not performing any dissection of the midface through the lower eyelid. The transtemporal approach was used to elevate the periosteum from the zygomatic arch and the superior aspect of the zygoma. The transoral approach was used to free the periosteum from the maxilla and inferior aspects of the zygoma. This combined approach had the advantage of allowing the surgeon a direct access for performing a subperiosteal dissection of the entire midface under direct vision without

the need of an endoscope. It also avoided the risk of lower eyelid retraction or ectropion (**Fig. 2**).

Whether superior movement of the midface soft tissues is accomplished by a deep plane, subperiosteal, or extended supra-SMAS facelift, the goal is to produce a dramatic lifting of midface tissues. Proponents of the extended supra-SMAS approach argue that the periosteum does not stretch with age and a subperiosteal approach repositions the origin of the zygomatic musculature to a more superior and abnormal position. This may have the affect of giving an excessive horizontal width to the midface. Considerably more postoperative facial edema is associated with this approach compared with the transfacial supra-SMAS dissection or the deep plane facelift. Another disadvantage of a subperiosteal dissection is that most approaches call for elevation of the periosteum from the anterior portion of the zygomatic arch, placing the temporal branch of the facial nerve at risk.

Proponents of the subperiosteal approach point to the safety of keeping all of the soft tissue including the facial nerve above the plane of dissection. There is less risk of injury to the zygomatic and buccal branches of the facial nerve using the subperiosteal approach compared with the deep plane or extended supra-SMAS facelift. There is no disruption of the blood supply to the skin of the midface because the plane of dissection is beneath all of the major blood supply to the face. There is no need for a lengthy skin flap lifted from the preauricular area, or for a blind dissection of soft tissues of the midface. The lower periocular area is maximally rejuvenated when mid-facelifting is performed in conjunction with orbicularis occuli repositioning to a more superior and medial position.[10] Repositioning of the ptotic orbicularis muscle is most easily accomplished by performing a subperiosteal mid-facelift. Although the composite rhytidectomy described by Hamra does reposition this muscle, supra-SMAS mid-facelifts do not. **Table 1** summarizes the advantages and disadvantages of the various approaches to lifting the midface.[9]

The extreme interest in developing new surgical approaches to rhytidectomy and to refining those techniques over the last two decades has resulted in considerable improvement in surgical results. This has taken the form of a more natural and youthful restoration of the face by together lifting forehead, midface, and lower face. This approach produces a more harmonious balance of the upper and lower portions of the face than was possible before the introduction of mid-facelifting techniques. Added to this has been the emphasis by

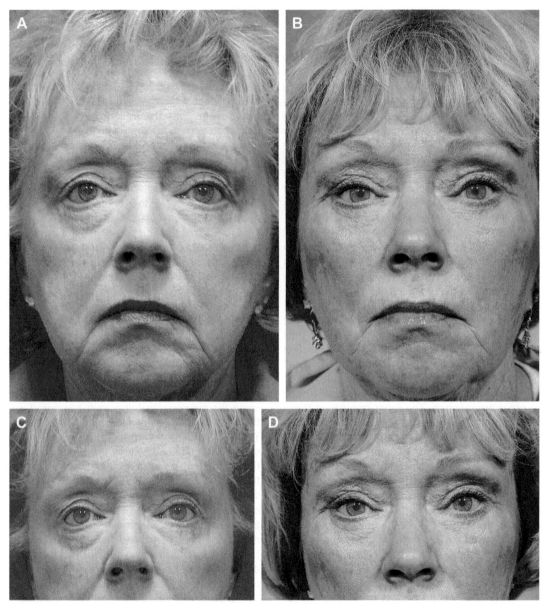

Fig. 2. (*A–D*) Preoperative and 6-month postoperative views. A subperiosteal mid-facelift was performed through a combined transoral and transtemporal approach. A drill hole canthoplasty was performed bilaterally concomitant with mid-facelift to correct lower eyelid ectropia.

some surgeons of restoring tissue volume to the face by using autogenous fat injections.[19] One can conclude that the most favorable results in face lifting occur when the lower cheek is rejuvenated by dissecting beneath the SMAS to create an advancement flap together with the lifting of the cheek fat of the midface posterosuperiorly. An alternative to mid-facelifting may be autogenous fat transfer to the midface. When performing fat injection of the face, it is necessary to overfill the midface because approximately two thirds of the transferred fat does not survive.[20]

SURGICAL APPROACHES

Although there are a multitude of variations in performing a rhytidectomy of the lower face and upper neck they may be divided into four categories according to the tissue planes used for dissection: (1) subcutaneous, (2) sub-SMAS, (3) supra-SMAS, and (4) subperiosteal.

Subcutaneous Rhytidectomy

All approaches except the endoscopic facelift without periauricular incisions call for some

Table 1
Dissection planes of mid-facelifting

	Advantages	Disadvantages
Subperiosteal	Does not require preauricular incision/skin flap Does not impair vascular supply of facial skin Avoids risk to zygomatic branch of VII nerve Lifts orbicularis occuli of lower eyelid Some lifting of oral commissure	Increases horizontal width of face Risk to temporal and buccal branches of VII nerve and infraorbital nerve Greater postoperative edema May cause hypesthesia of malar eminence
Supra-SMAS	Does not reposition zygomatic musculature Avoids risk to temporal and buccal branches of VII nerve Risk to zygomatic branch of VII nerve	Long preauricular cutaneous flap Reduces skin vascularity of face Less postoperative edema Does not lift orbicularis occuli

From Baker SR. Rhytidectomy. In: Cummings CW, Flint PW, Harker LA, et al, editors. Otolaryngology-head and neck surgery, vol. 1. Philadelphia: Elsevier; 2008.

subcutaneous tissue dissection of the facial skin. The postauricular skin flap is always elevated in the subcutaneous tissue plane. Likewise, the preauricular skin must be dissected in the subcutaneous tissue plane for variable distances before incisions can be made through the SMAS. Typically, the skin of the upper neck is also elevated in the subcutaneous tissue plane or immediately superficial to the platysmal muscle (preplatysmal). Dissection may continue forward in the neck to the midline. The extent of anterior dissection in the subcutaneous tissue plane of the face is dependent on the surgeon's preference and may be influenced by the degree of facial skin laxity. In the past, there have been controversies concerning the benefits of long versus short flap rhytidectomies. A benefit of dissecting to the lateral bony orbital rim in the temple is that it releases the skin from the underlying orbicularis occuli. This helps to improve the crow's feet and also assists with redistribution of the vertically advanced preauricular skin flap. Once a skin flap has been elevated, the exposed SMAS can be imbricated by folding it on itself using sutures to suspend it to the periparotid fascia. The subcutaneous facelift with imbrication of the SMAS is still the most common surgical approach used by plastic surgeons, composing 23% of facelift procedures performed.[21] It is probably the safest approach from the standpoint of risk of facial nerve injury, but has the disadvantages compared with other techniques of shorter long-term improvement of the jowl and no correction of the midface. A technique advocated by Little[22] involves an extended

anterior subcutaneous tissue dissection of the lower cheek from the ear to the upper lip. The exposed SMAS and cheek fat is then suture suspended vertically using multiple interrupted sutures. This elevates the jowl and oral commissure superiorly. The approach has the advantage of moving ptotic cheek fat located in the area of the jowl toward the submalar region. This in turn increases the tissue volume in submalar region of the face providing a more rounded contour of the midface. This is particularly advantageous in patients displaying submalar wasting associated with aging. The greatest disadvantage of the extended subcutaneous facelift dissection is the long preauricular skin flap resulting from a lengthy anterior dissection. This creates a potentially large dead space in which hematomas and seromas may collect.

Superficial Musculoaponeurotic System Rhytidectomy

The sub-SMAS dissection of the lower face is another common surgical approach performed by approximately 20% of facelift surgeons.[21] This may take the form of elevating a SMAS flap limited to the area over the parotid gland (25% of surgeons) or extending the SMAS flap anterior to the parotid gland. The SMAS flap is then suspended posterosuperiorly. Neither of these approaches lifts the midface but they markedly improve the jowl. When a SMAS flap is dissected from the parotid fascia, it is frequently referred to as a "SMAS rhytidectomy." Dissecting beneath the SMAS anterior to the parotid gland and then transitioning to a supra-SMAS plane and dissecting all of the cheek fat with attached overlying skin away from the zygomatic musculature as described by Hamra[8] is known as a "deep plane rhytidectomy." Later, Hamra added to this dissection a supraperiosteal dissection of the superior aspect of the midface through a lower eyelid incision. This biplane dissection was termed a "composite rhytidectomy" by Hamra.[10] Nine percent of facelift surgeons perform a deep plane or composite rhytidectomy.[21]

A variation of the sub-SMAS dissection is a strip SMASectomy described by Baker.[23] This technique consists of excising a strip of SMAS along a line that extends from the angle of the mandible to the lateral malar eminence. Usually a 2 to 4 cm wide strip of SMAS is excised depending on laxity. Much of this excision is anterior to the parotid gland. No anterior dissection beneath the SMAS is performed. The SMAS is reapproximated advancing the mobile SMAS and platysma posterosuperior to the junction of the SMAS fixed to the periparotid fascia. Approximately 20% of facelift surgeons use the technique of SMASectomy.[21] It has the advantage of simplicity but does not address the midface.

Suprasuperficial Musculoaponeurotic System Rhytidectomy

The term "supra-SMAS" usually refers to dissection just superficial to the SMAS in the midface. All subcutaneous dissections in the preauricular area are also supra-SMAS. Remaining just superficial to the SMAS as the limits of the dissection are extended anteriorly beyond the parotid gland toward the midface, however, requires a deeper dissection than is required for a standard subcutaneous facelift or the technique described by Little.[22] Because the SMAS invests the mimetic muscles of the midface, a supra-SMAS dissection requires a forward dissection immediately superficial to these muscles. This results in a thick cutaneous flap consisting of cheek fat and overlying attached facial skin. The dissection is usually carried to the upper lip to release all of the dermal attachments of the SMAS to the melolabial crease. This extreme anterior dissection is commonly referred to as an "extended SMAS rhytidectomy" or an "extended supra-SMAS rhytidectomy." The cutaneous flap is then suspended under considerable tension posterosuperiorly to the fascia overlying zygoma and parotid gland. The primary purpose of the extended supra-SMAS rhytidectomy is to displace superiorly the cheek fat of the midface. This corrects the ptotic cheek fat that

occurs in the midface with aging and softens the melolabial fold.

The main disadvantage of the extended supra-SMAS rhytidectomy is the long preauricular skin flap resulting from a lengthy anterior dissection. This creates a potentially large dead space in which hematomas may collect. A dissection beyond the convexity of the zygoma may require some blind dissection or at least impair the exposure available to the surgeon. In addition, remaining above the SMAS throughout the dissection does not provide as much improvement of the jowl compared with developing a SMAS flap of the inferior cheek. Approximately 20% of facelift surgeons perform the extended supra-SMAS rhytidectomy.[21] The advantage of the deep plane facelift compared with the supra-SMAS lift is that the inferior cheek is dissected in a sub-SMAS plane creating an advancement flap, whereas the midface is dissected in a supra-SMAS plane. The sub-SMAS dissection in the lower face provides long-term correction of the jowl.[24]

Subperiosteal Rhytidectomy

Subperiosteal rhytidectomy refers to the lifting of the cheek tissues by dissecting in the subperiosteal plane over the maxilla and zygoma. The procedure also usually includes an endoscopic subperiosteal forehead lift. All of the soft tissues of the midface are lifted including the elevators of the lip, the zygomatic major and minor, and often the orbicularis occuli. The fundamental difference between the subperiosteal mid-facelift and the transfacial supra-SMAS facelift is the superior displacement of these muscles. The extended supra-SMAS and deep plane rhytidectomy only elevate the cheek fat and skin and not the muscles of the midface. Subperiosteal mid-facelifts do not significantly correct the jowl and have no influence on the upper neck. Another disadvantage of a subperiosteal mid-facelift is the tendency to increase the horizontal width of the face by displacing the origin of the zygomatic major muscle to a more superior and lateral position. In most patients, however, this has the pleasing effect of enhancing the malar eminence.

There are four surgical approaches used to perform subperiosteal mid-facelifting: (1) transtemporal usually using an endoscope, (2) transorbital through a lower eyelid or transconjunctival incision, (3) transoral through an upper gingival buccal incision, and (4) combined using two or more of the previously listed approaches. Regardless of the approach, it is necessary to release the periosteum from the lateral and inferior bony orbital rim and from the entire zygoma and maxilla.

Table 2
Surgical approaches to mid-facelifting

Surgical Approach	Plane of Dissection	Advantages	Disadvantages
Transfacial	Supra-SMAS	Avoids risk to temporal and buccal branches of VII nerve Less postoperative edema	Preauricular incision and long skin flap Requires some blind dissection Does not lift orbicularis occuli
Transtemporal	Subperiosteal	No preauricular incision Concomitant lateral brow lift	Risk to temporal and buccal branches of VII nerve Requires endoscope Poor access to periosteal dissection of maxilla
Transorbital	Subperiosteal or supraperiosteal	Direct access for dissection and suspension of midface More vertical vector for suspension of midface soft tissues	Risk to buccal branch of VII nerve Risk to infraorbital nerve Risk of lower lid retraction/ectropion
Transoral	Subperiosteal	Direct access for dissection of midface Ease in elevating periosteum of maxilla	Risk to buccal branch of VII nerve Does not provide access for suspension of midface tissues Greater risk of infection Risk to infraorbital nerve
Combined	Subperiosteal usually transoral combined with transtemporal or transorbital	Direct visualization of entire dissection Ease of suspension of midface tissues	More postoperative edema Greater risk of infection if transoral route used

From Baker SR. Rhytidectomy. In: Cummings CW, Flint PW, Harker LA, et al, editors. Otolaryngology-head and neck surgery, vol. 1. Philadelphia: Elsevier; 2008.

The temporal approach is accomplished through an incision behind the hairline in the temple. An endoscope is frequently used to perform a dissection beneath the temporoparietal fascia of the anterior lateral scalp. Transition is then made to a subperiosteal plane as dissection continues inferiorly over the zygoma and zygomatic arch. Subperiosteal dissection also proceeds medially in the midface releasing the soft tissues from their attachment to the maxilla. This necessitates limited dissection onto the upper portion of the masseter muscle. A disadvantage of the transtemporal approach is the difficulty releasing the periosteum from the medial maxilla because of insufficient exposure even when an endoscope is used.

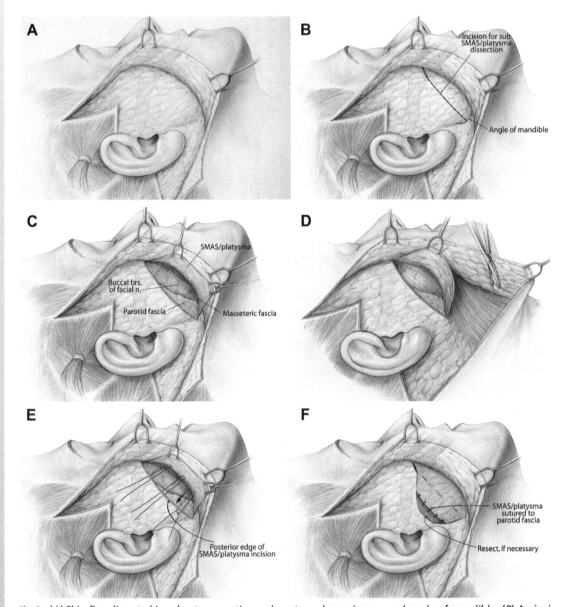

Fig. 3. (A) Skin flap dissected in subcutaneous tissue plane to malar eminence and angle of mandible. (B) An incision is made through the SMAS from malar eminence to angle of mandible. (C) SMAS platysmal flap dissected superficial to masseteric fascia anteriorly beneath jowl. Branches of the facial nerve remain deep to masseteric fascia. (D) SMAS flap dissected anteriorly. Neck skin dissected to midline in preplatysmal plane. Excess subcutaneous fat removed from neck flap. (E) SMAS flap suspended by sewing deep aspect of elevated platysma to the posterior incise border of the SMAS. (F) SMAS platysma flap overlapping parotid gland sutured to periparotid fascia to reinforce suspension of SMAS. (Figs. B and E From Baker SR. Triplane rhytidectomy combining the best of all worlds. Arch Otol Head Neck Surg 1997;123:1167–72.)

The transorbital route has the advantage of direct access to the midface with less need for the use of an endoscope. Through this approach, the subperiosteal dissection is accomplished under direct vision and the midface soft tissues are suspended either to the inferior bony orbital rim or to the anteroinferior temporalis fascia. Some surgeons perform a supraperiosteal dissection of the midface through a lower eyelid incision. A disadvantage of the transorbital approach is temporary distortion of the lateral canthal area from bunching of redundant soft tissue. Another disadvantage is the risk of lower eyelid retraction or ectropion.

The transoral approach is not often used by itself, but is combined with transorbital or transtemporal incisions to create a combined surgical approach.[25,26] This enables the periosteum to be easily stripped from the inferior aspects of the maxilla and zygoma from the oral access. The remaining periosteum is then elevated from the superior aspect of the zygoma and from the anterior zygomatic arch through an orbital or temporal access. The advantage of this combined approach is ease of dissection and direct visualization without the need for an endoscope. The main disadvantage is the potential risk of wound infection because of exposure of the dissection to bacteria in the oral cavity. **Table 2** summarizes the surgical approaches to the midface and the advantages and disadvantages of each.[9] Only 2% of facelift surgeons generally perform subperiosteal facelifting, and of those approximately half use an endoscope.[21]

SURGICAL TECHNIQUES

Regardless of the surgical approach used to perform a rhytidectomy, the goals are the same. These include (1) preserving motor and sensory innervation of the face, (2) modifying cervical fat if excessive, (3) tightening the SMAS and platysma, and (4) redraping cervical and facial skin and trim excess. This article has discussed many of the

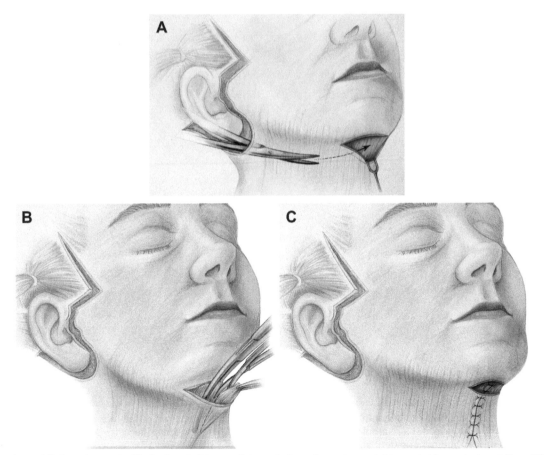

Fig. 4. (*A*) Superior neck skin is elevated in preplatysmal plane from sternocleidomastoid muscle to midline. (*B*) Redundant platysmal muscle resected vertically in midline of neck. (*C*) Incised borders of platysma approximated with interrupted sutures.

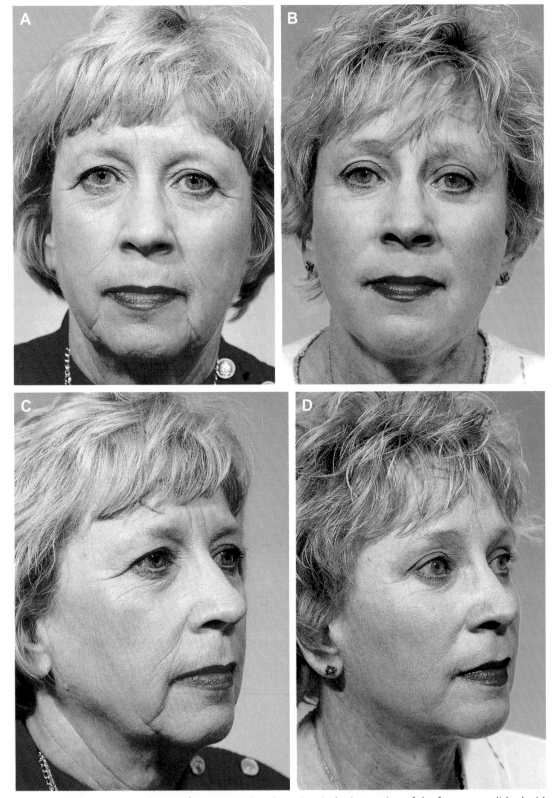

Fig. 5. (*A–F*) Preoperative and 6-month postoperative views. Surgical rejuvenation of the face accomplished with upper and lower eyelid blepharoplasty, subperiosteal mid-facelift, sub-SMAS facelift, submentoplasty as described in text, and perioral dermabrasion.

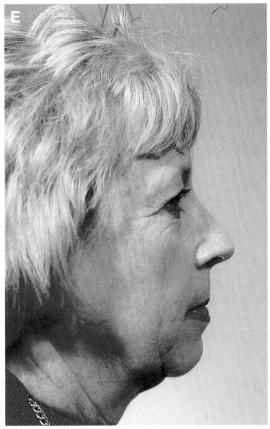

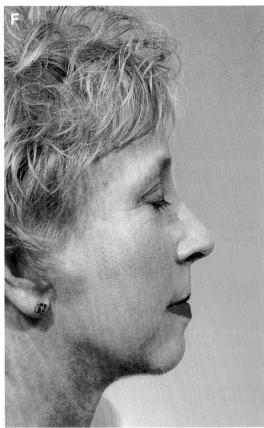

Fig. 5. (*continued*)

approaches used to achieve these goals and lists many of the advantages and disadvantages of each surgical approach. This section addresses more technical aspects of facelifting.

Skin Flap and Superficial Musculoaponeurotic System Elevation

The extent of skin undermining varies with each patient and the surgical approach used. When a sub-SMAS dissection is performed, the facial skin may be left attached to the underlying SMAS or may be separated from the portion of the SMAS dissected as a flap. Leaving the skin attached to the SMAS helps to preserve the integrity of this structure and facilitates an easier sub-SMAS dissection. It also provides more substance for suture suspension of the SMAS flap. The depth of dissection varies in each region of the face. The posterior scalp is elevated below the hair follicles transitioning to a more superficial subcutaneous tissue plane under the postauricular skin. Over the sternocleidomastoid muscle, the dissection must be very superficial remaining above the fascia of the muscle to avoid injury to the greater

auricular nerve. Anterior to the sternocleidomastoid muscle the neck skin is dissected either in the subcutaneous tissue plane or immediately superficial to the platysma. The preplatysmal plane is preferred by the author because it enables the surgeon to remove excessive fat accurately from the cervical skin flap.

In the temple, the dissection may be in the subgaleal plane or below the hair follicles in the deep subcutaneous tissue plane. The subcutaneous tissue plane is preferred to the subgaleal approach because greater lifting is possible of the skin lateral to the eye. If the subcutaneous tissue plane is used, the dissection should transition to a more superficial level under the temple skin anterior to the hairline.

Over the parotid gland in the preauricular area, dissection is accomplished in the subcutaneous tissue plane. The anterior extent of the dissection varies with the surgical approach used. **Fig. 3** shows a series of drawings that demonstrate the author's usual surgical approach to lifting the lower face.[25] The author extends the dissection forward to a line extending from the lateral canthus to the angle of the mandible. The dissection does

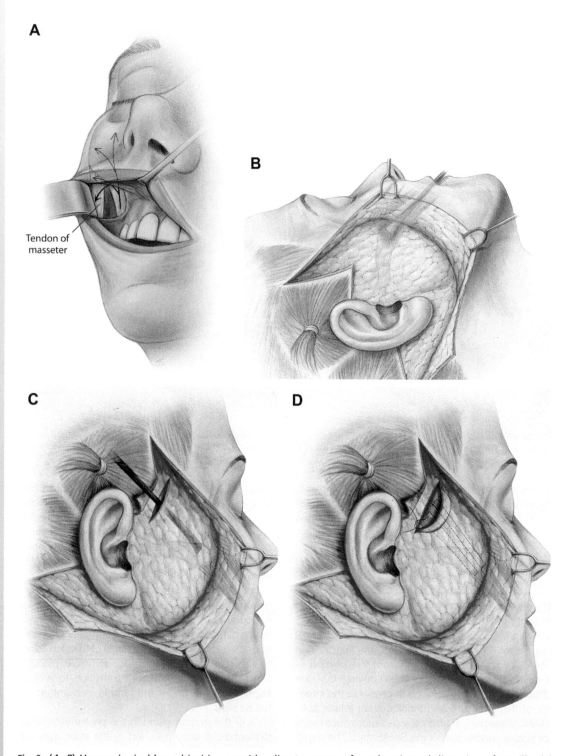

Fig. 6. (*A, B*) Upper gingival buccal incision provides direct exposure for subperiosteal dissection of maxilla. (*C*) The periosteum of the superior aspect of the zygoma, zygomatic bony arch, and frontal process of the zygoma is dissected through temporal incision remaining deep to the temporal parietal fascia. (*D*) Soft tissue of the midface freed from its bony attachments to the maxilla and zygoma is suspended to the temporalis fascia.

not extend beyond this line so as to leave the facial skin attached to the underlying SMAS. In individuals with marked laxity of the cervical skin or who require liposculpturing, a posterior neck dissection in the relatively avascular preplatysmal plane is carried forward from the upper sternocleidomastoid muscle to the midline. Lifting the cervical fat with the skin enables the surgeon to remove fat from the flap selectively and evenly under direct vision using scissors or a liposculpturing cannula.

Once the posterior neck dissection is completed, the SMAS is dissected by making an incision through the SMAS from the malar eminence to the angle of the mandible. The upper third of the incision is undermined 2 cm to allow a cuff of SMAS for suturing. The lower two thirds of the incision are undermined in the subplatysmal plane. The dissection is carried forward beneath the jowl, remaining above the inferior border of the mandible and deep to the platysma. This is accomplished with ease, primarily by blunt dissection because the SMAS-platysma is separated in this region from the masseter muscle and buccal fat by a layer of loose areolar tissue between the platysma and the masseter fascia. The dissection must remain superficial to the masseteric fascia because the facial nerve lies deep to the fascia (see **Fig. 3**). If a classical deep plane facelift as described by Hamra[8] is planned, attention is now turned toward dissection of the midface fat. Dissection of the midface is commenced at the malar eminence. Remaining immediately superficial to the zygomatic muscle, the cheek fat with attached overlying skin is mobilized away from the zygomatic musculature primarily by blunt dissection, which extends medially to the modiolus of the lip commissure and beneath the melolabial fold to its junction with the upper lip. Once this tissue plane has been developed, it is connected to the sub-SMAS plane by lifting upward on both areas of dissection with elevators and then sharply connecting the two individual tissue planes, releasing the SMAS from its midface attachments (see **Fig. 1**). This maneuver creates a single thick facial flap consisting of cheek skin and underlying platysma and midface fat. Before advancement of the SMAS and the midface fat (if a deep plane facelift has been completed) the cervical skin flap is liposculptured by removing excessive subcutaneous fat from the cervical skin flap. The SMAS is suspended posterosuperiorly following suspension of the midface, if a deep plane or subperiosteal mid-facelift has been performed. Sutures are placed through the ventral aspect of the elevated platysma of the inferior cheek and secured to the posterior incised border of the SMAS. This causes marked posterosuperior advancement of the SMAS flap, the advance border of which overlaps the parotid gland and is secured to the preauricular parotid fascia with a second series of suspension sutures. The SMAS flap is often advanced to within 2 cm of the earlobe, and on occasion may require excision and discarding of redundant SMAS and platysmal muscle. The advancement produces a short skin flap in this area.

Submentoplasty

Ellenbogen and Karlin[27] have established five visual criteria that the eye translates as a youthful profile of the neck: (1) distinct inferior mandibular border from mentum to angle with no jowl overhang; (2) slight subhyoid depression at the apex of the cervicomental angle, which depression on profile gives the impression of a thin and long neck; (3) visible thyroid cartilage convexity; (4) distinct visible anterior border of the sternocleidomastoid muscle in its entire length from mastoid to sternum; and (5) cervicomental angle between 105 and 120 degrees. This translates into a 90-degree angle between the axis of the sternocleidomastoid muscle and a line drawn tangent to the submentum in an anteroposterior orientation.[27] An inferior positioned hyoid, excessive submental fat, laxity of the platysma (anterior bands), and microgenia can all contribute to blunting of the cervicomental angle.

Anterior bands that develop near the midline of the neck with age are the result of elastosis and sagging of the platysmal muscles. When banding is mild, they can be eradicated by developing a platysmal flap posterior near the angle of the mandible and advancing this flap posterosuperior

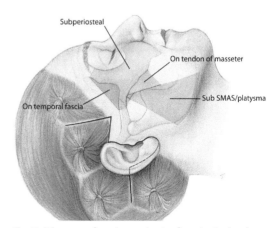

Fig. 7. Diagram showing extent of periosteal release from the midface bony structures and the extent of sub-SMAS dissection typically performed by the author.

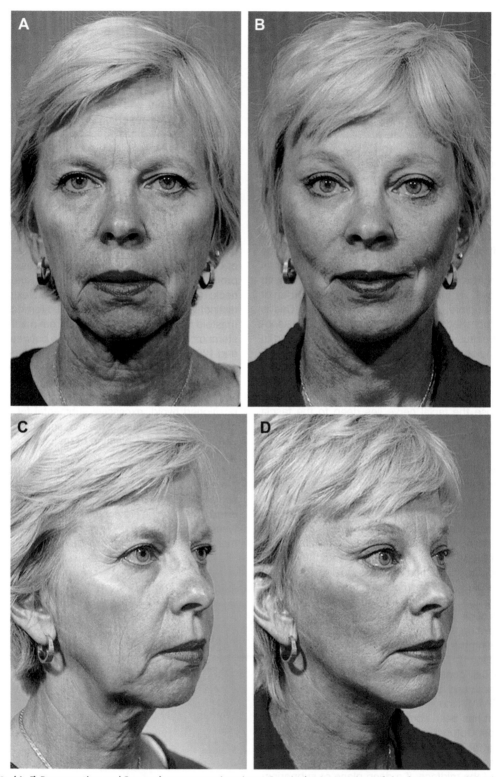

Fig. 8. (*A–F*) Preoperative and 3-month postoperative views. Surgical rejuvenation of the face accomplished with endoscopic forehead lift, subperiosteal mid-facelift, and sub-SMAS facelift. Note enhancement of malar eminence from lifting midface.

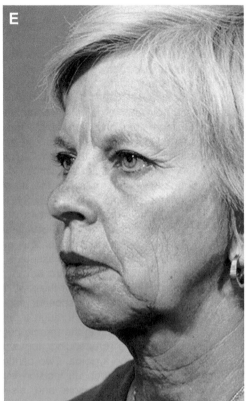

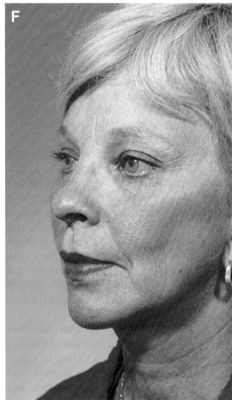

Fig. 8. (*continued*)

over the parotid gland. Another less effective method is to suture suspend the lateral border of the muscle below the angle of the mandible to the fascia of the mastoid and sternocleidomastoid muscle. In the past, surgeons advocated partial or complete horizontal division of the platysmal muscle 5 cm or more below the mandible to achieve a greater posterior advancement of the muscle flap and better topographic delineation between the neck and the lower jaw. This practice has been abandoned because of unnatural contours and deformities that develop in the neck as a result of this technique.

When managing platysmal bands, the most effective method, with greatest longevity of results, is to correct the deformity anteriorly where it is located. This is accomplished by performing a submentoplasty. A submentoplasty is indicated if the patient has excessive fatty deposits in the submental area, marked elastosis of neck skin, or platysmal banding. The author performs a submentoplasty with or without posterior neck dissection in a manner described by Hamra (**Fig. 4**).[8] A submentoplasty is required in most patients having rhytidectomy and typically is the first stage of a rhytidectomy. A 2.5-cm curvilinear incision is made just anterior to the submental crease. A

flap consisting of skin and all of the fat superficial to the platysmal muscle is elevated in a preplatysmal plane. This dissection extends to the level of the superior aspect of the thyroid cartilage and laterally for 6 cm on either side of midline. In the paramedian position, the platysmal muscles are bluntly undermined in a vertical direction from the mandible to the level of the thyroid cartilage and then cross-clamped and incised. The muscle between the two incisions is resected. The amount of muscle removed depends on redundancy. Sufficient muscle should be removed so that when the borders of the two platysmal muscles are brought together, tautness is created. Before suturing the muscles together, any excess subplatysmal fat is resected under direct vision. The incised borders of the platysmal muscles are then approximated with interrupted sutures burying the knot beneath the muscles (see **Fig. 4**). Any excess fat elevated with the submental skin is removed with scissors under direct vision. Other surgeons prefer to use suction-assisted liposculpturing to modify the submental fat instead of direct excision using scissors. Sixty percent of facelift surgeons perform direct excision of submental fat, whereas only 27% perform suction-assisted lipectomy.[21] Perhaps the reason for the popularity of direct excision is that a greater amount of subcutaneous fat can be removed with greater ease and accuracy using direct excision compared with the use of a suction cannula. Because the skin of the neck is attached to the platysmal muscle, wide undermining of the skin in the submental area is necessary to prevent bunching of the submental skin when the platysma is advanced medially. This is the greatest disadvantage of a submentoplasty as described.

Some surgeons prefer to perform a horizontal incision of the platysma extending laterally from its anterior border for variable distances at the level of the thyroid cartilage. The two platysmal muscles are then sutured together in the midline without excision of muscle tissue. The horizontal incision is believed by some to create a more acute cervicomental angle. Transecting the muscle and midline suturing is performed by 40% of surgeons, whereas 21% perform vertical incision and resection of the platysmal redundancy and midline suturing.[21]

The advantage of resecting redundant platysmal muscle is the elimination of the excess muscle and subplatysmal fat rather than attempting to imbricate the redundancy. By resecting muscle and advancing the platysma medially toward the midline, the surgeon is addressing the deformity at its origin and is advancing tissue in the same direction as the gravitational forces on the neck. This approach provides a pleasing, youthful anterior neck contour (**Fig. 5**). In contrast, posterior suspension of the platysma near the angle of the mandible is removed from the area of deformity and moves tissue against gravitational pull. Posterior suspension of the cervical platysma is frequently prone to early recurrence of banding.

Even with the direct approach of correcting banding by performing a surgical excision of muscle redundancy, the anterior neck is the weak link of facelifting. Relaxation of skin and platysma occurs here first before other areas of the face and neck. Mild recurrent banding and skin laxity of the submentum may be observed as soon as 6 months following facelifting. This may be related to the increased tissue creep observe in the SMAS located in the neck compared with the SMAS in the cheek.[28] Patients should be counseled that anterior neck laxity and melolabial folds are the two regions of the face that are most difficult to correct completely with rhytidectomy.

Subperiosteal Mid-facelift

If a subperiosteal mid-facelift is to be performed, this is accomplished before dissecting SMAS flaps. A sub-SMAS dissection does not improve the midface. The author usually performs a subperiosteal mid-facelift through a combined transoral and transtemporal approach (**Fig. 6**). Bilateral subperiosteal midface dissection is accomplished under direct vision using a headlight and tissue retractor. A 2-cm upper gingival buccal incision is made and with the use of a periosteal elevator a complete detachment of the periosteum from the face of the maxilla is accomplished including release from the pyriform aperture, nasal sidewall, the entire infraorbital bony rim, and zygomatic eminence. Care is taken to observe and preserve the infraorbital nerve. From the zygoma, the dissection is carried inferiorly over the anterior masseter for 2 cm, releasing the soft tissue from its attachment to the anterior tendonous aspect of the muscle. This maneuver detaches the masseteric cutaneous ligaments, allowing upward advancement of the platysma in the region of the jowl.[11] Subperiosteal dissection of the superior aspect of the zygoma is accomplished through a temporal scalp incision. Dissection in the temple begins in the subgaleal plane proceeding forward and downward toward the zygoma. Two centimeters above the zygomatic arch an incision is made through the temporalis fascia and dissection continues just superficial to the temporal fat pad to the level of the medial aspect of the zygomatic arch. An incision is then made through the periosteum along the superior border of the arch and the periosteum is raised off of the arch. Dissection of the subperiosteal plane continues anteriorly to connect with the dissection plane created from the transoral approach. The periosteum is also elevated off of the frontal process of the zygoma to free the periosteum from the entire lateral orbital bony rim. **Fig. 7** diagrams the extent of periosteal release from the midface bony structures and the extent of sub-SMAS dissection typically performed by the author. Once all of the soft tissue of the midface has been freed from its bony attachment to the maxilla and zygoma, the tissue is suspended with sutures placed between the periosteum overlying the malar eminence and the temporalis fascia. This suspension is placed under considerable tension. Marked upward movement of the soft tissues is noted often resulting in exposure of the upper incisors. Suspension of the midface soft tissues is always performed before suspension of the SMAS flap. Subperiosteal mid-facelifts reposition the ptotic cheek fat to a more youthful position. It also lifts the orbicularis muscle of the lower eyelid and restores the relationship between the lower eyelid and the cheek observed in youthful faces (**Fig. 8**).

SUMMARY

Surgical approaches to rhytidectomy and to refining those techniques over the last two decades have resulted in considerable improvement in surgical outcomes. This has resulted in a more natural and youthful restoration of the face by together lifting forehead, midface and lower face. This comprehensive approach to facial rejuvenation has produced a more harmonious balance of the upper and lower portions of the face than was possible before the introduction of mid-facelifting techniques. Adding to these techniques has been the emphasis by some surgeons of restoring tissue volume to the face using autogenous fat grafting. It is evident that the most favorable results in facelifting occur when the lower cheek is rejuvenated by dissecting beneath the musculoaponeurotic system to create an advancement flap together with the lifting of the cheek fat of the midface posterosuperior.

REFERENCES

1. Rogers BO. History of the development of aesthetic surgery. In: Regnault P, Daniel RK, editors. Aesthetic plastic surgery. Boston/Toronto: Little, Brown and Company; 1984.
2. Skoog TG. Plastic surgery: the aging face. In: Skoog TG, editor. Plastic surgery: new methods and refinements. Philadelphia: W.B. Saunders; 1974.
3. Mitz V, Peyronie M. The superficial musculo-aponeurotic system (SMAS) in the parotid and cheek area. Plast Reconstr Surg 1976;58:80–8.
4. Yousif NJ, Gosain A, Matloub HS, et al. The nasolabial fold: an anatomic and histologic reappraisal. Plast Reconstr Surg 1994;93:60–9.
5. Barton FE Jr. The SMAS and the nasolabial fold. Plast Reconstr Surg 1992;89:1054–7.
6. Gassner HG, Rafii A, Young A, et al. Surgical anatomy of the face: implications for modern facelift techniques. Arch Facial Plast Surg 2008;10(1):9–19.
7. Barton FE Jr. Rhytidectomy and the nasolabial fold. Plast Reconstr Surg 1992;90:601–7.
8. Hamra ST. The deep-plane rhytidectomy. Plast Reconstr Surg 1990;86:53–61.
9. Baker SR. Rhytidectomy. In: Cummings CW, Flint PW, Harker LA, et al, editors, Otolaryngology: head and neck surgery, vol. 1. Philadelphia: Elsevier; 2005. p. 714–49.
10. Hamra ST. Composite rhytidectomy. Plast Reconstr Surg 1992;90:1–13.
11. Owsley JQ. Lifting the malar fat pad for correction of prominent nasolabial folds. Plast Reconstr Surg 1993;91:463–74.
12. Tessier F. Facelifting and frontal rhytidectomy. In: Ely TF, editor. Transactions of the Seventh International Congress of plastic and reconstructive surgery. Rio de Janeiro: Sociedade Brasileira de Cirurgia Plastica; 1980. p. 33.
13. Psillakis JM, Rumley TO, Camargos A. Subperiosteal approach as an improved concept for correction of the aging face. Plast Reconstr Surg 1988; 82:383–92.
14. Ramirez OM, Maillard GF, Musolas A. The extended subperiosteal facelift: a definitive soft-tissue remodeling for facial rejuvenation. Plast Reconstr Surg 1991;88:227–36.
15. Paul MD. The perosteal hinge flap in the superiosteal cheek-lift. Oper Tech Plast Reconstr Surg 1998;5(2): 145–54.
16. Gunter JP, Hackney FL. A simplified transblepharoplasty subperiosteal cheek lift. Plast Reconstr Surg 1999;103(7):2029–35.
17. Hester TR, Codner MA, McCord CD, et al. Evolution of technique of the direct transblepharoplasty approach for the correction of lower lid and midfacial aging: maximizing results and minimizing complications in a 5-year experience. Plast Reconstr Surg 2000;105(1):393–406.
18. Hester TR, Codner MA, McCord CD, et al. Transorbital lower-lid and midface rejuvenation. Oper Tech Plast Reconstr Surg 1998;5:163–83.
19. Coleman SR. Facial recontouring with lipostructure. Clin Plast Surg 1997;24:347–67.
20. Meier JD, Glasgold RA, Glasgold MJ. Autologous fat grafting long-term evidence of its efficacy in midfacial rejuvenation. Arch Facial Plast Surg 2009; 11(1):24–8.
21. Matarasso A, Elkwood A, Rankin M, et al. National plastic surgery survey: facelift techniques and complications. Plast Reconstr Surg 2000;106(5): 1185–95.
22. Little JW. Three-dimensional rejuvenation of the midface: volumetric resculpture by malar imbrication. Plast Reconstr Surg 2000;105:267–85.
23. Baker DC. Lateral SMASectomy. Plast Reconstr Surg 1997;100(2):509–13.
24. Hamra ST. A study of the long-term effect of malar fat repositioning in face lift surgery: short-term success but long-term failure. Plast Reconstr Surg 2002;110(3):940–51.
25. Baker SR. Triplane rhytidectomy: combining the best of all worlds. Arch Otolaryngol Head Neck Surg 1997;123:1167–72.
26. Baker SR. Multiplane rhytidectomy. Oper Tech Otolaryngol Head Neck Surg 1999;10(3):184–91.
27. Ellenbogen R, Karlin JV. Visual criteria for success in restoring the youthful neck. Plast Reconstr Surg 1980;66(6):826–37.
28. Har-Shai Y, Bodner SR, Egozy-Golan D, et al. Mechanical properties and microstructure of the superficial musculoaponeurotic system. Plast Reconstr Surg 1996;98(1):59–70.

Extended Superficial Muscular Aponeurotic System Rhytidectomy: A Graded Approach

Stephen W. Perkins, MD*, Amit B. Patel, MD

KEYWORDS

- Rhytidectomy • Facelift • SMAS-Facelift
- Aging face • Facial rejuvenation

The acceptance of rhytidectomy has been a relatively recent phenomenon. Until the twentieth century, aesthetic surgery was shrouded in secrecy, and well into the twentieth century prominent physicians often were guarded in sharing their experience, despite rumors of cosmetic surgery taking place in private offices and clinics. After World War II, Fomon came to prominence as one of the founders and leaders of the American Academy of Facial Plastic and Reconstructive Surgery. Fomon willingly taught cosmetic surgery to those who were interested. One of his contributions was his recognition of the limits of subcutaneous rhytidectomy: "The average duration of the beneficial effects, even with the best technical skill, cannot be expected to exceed three to four years".[1]

By the 1960s and 1970s, advances in anesthesia allowed elective surgery to be performed safely. Cosmetic surgery literally came out of the dark ages by embracing the free exchange of ideas between surgeons, critical analysis of short- and long-term results by a peer-reviewed scientific community, and the growing need to accommodate a rapidly growing aging population.

The baby-boom generation brought a new era in facial plastic and reconstructive surgery. A major advance in the approach to rhytidectomy came in 1974 when Skoog[2] published his thoughts on subfascial rhytidectomy. In 1976, Mitz and Peyronie[3] described this subfascial layer anatomically as the superficial muscular aponeurotic system (SMAS). Skoog and Lemmon[4] demonstrated that by undermining and moving SMAS, the entire skin and SMAS unit moved together as a "the sliding tectonic plate." This approach was the first advocating the effectiveness of imbrication (advancement, shortening, and suturing) as a technique in rhytidectomy.

The search for a natural looking rhytidectomy with longer-lasting results continued into the 1980s. Webster demonstrated that simply plicating (pulling back, folding over, and suturing) the underlying fascia and muscular layer often gave a nice, if not equal, improvement in the jaw and neckline, thereby achieving a natural appearance with few complications.[1]

Emphasis turned to improving the midface, traditionally the most difficult region of the face to rejuvenate surgically. The deep-plane and composite rhytidectomy were the next step in the evolution of facelift. These techniques were pioneered by Hamra[5] and seemed to achieve improvement in the nasolabial fold region. Other surgeons have concurred that these techniques produce improved results.[6]

Surgical approaches for rhytidectomy continue to evolve. From conservative skin flap elevations to the bi- and triplane rhytidectomy of Baker[7] to the deep-plane techniques of Kamer[6] and the subperiosteal dissections of Ramirez,[8] the literature demonstrates significant differences of opinion in managing the aging face. A balance must be drawn between extended operative times, duration of postoperative healing, level of assumed risk and complications, and durability of results. Over the past 26 years, the senior author has

Meridian Plastic Surgeons, 170 W. 106th Street, Indianapolis, IN 46290, USA
* Corresponding author.
E-mail address: sperkins@meridianplastic.com (S.W. Perkins).

Facial Plast Surg Clin N Am 17 (2009) 575–587
doi:10.1016/j.fsc.2009.06.008
1064-7406/09/$ – see front matter © 2009 Published by Elsevier Inc.

used a graded approach in combination with the modified deep-plane facelift that has consistently achieved natural-appearing results and satisfied patients. This article outlines the analysis of the patient, preoperative preparation of the patient, an algorithm for adjunctive procedures to achieve a youthful yet balanced face, surgical technique, and possible complications.

PREOPERATIVE CONSIDERATIONS
Consultation in Facelift

It is imperative that the preoperative consultation process represent a reciprocated balance of communication between the surgeon and the patient. In an era in which the term "facial rejuvenation" spans a variety of treatments ranging from botulinum toxin injections to deep-plane rhytidectomy, the goals of surgery can be lost in translation, with postoperative dissatisfaction quick to follow. It therefore is important both that the patient quickly understands the surgeon's philosophy and has a realistic expectation of what a facelift can and cannot accomplish and that the surgeon understands the patient's motivation for surgery. Patients who want to "look as young as they feel" or who are motivated to undergo surgery to enhance their self-esteem often seem to benefit from surgery. This high level of satisfaction is not seen as consistently with patients who do not have realistic expectations of surgery, who might be pressured to have surgery by a relative or spouse, who are mentally or emotionally unstable, or who believe that the surgery will solve a failing marriage. It is important to be alert for these red flags and to listen to the ancillary staffs' concerns. Patients often reveal their true motivations when the surgeon is not present. When the surgeon is unsure of the patient's motivation, the patient should be brought back for a second consultation.

The patient also needs to complete a detailed report of his or her medical history, which then is reviewed thoroughly to screen for conditions that may place the individual at a higher risk for complications from an elective surgery. It also is worthwhile to note diseases that might prolong the postoperative healing time. These conditions include diabetes, peripheral vascular disease, collagen vascular diseases, and some autoimmune disorders. It also is very important to identify any patient who is actively smoking. Smoking greatly compromises the vasculature of the skin flap, increasing the likelihood of postoperative necrosis and sloughing. Therefore, the authors often elect not to perform rhytidectomy in someone who is actively smoking; at the very least, they perform a shorter skin flap elevation. Any laser resurfacing over the area of skin undermining also should be staged no sooner than 2 months after surgery. Patients who chose smoking cessation should avoid all forms of tobacco and nicotine, including the nicotine patch, for at least 1 week before surgery and for 2 weeks after surgery. Frequently, medications such as buproprion, diazepam, or varenicline are prescribed to help combat withdrawal side effects and cravings.

Patients who have undergone a full course of head and neck radiation can have microvascular compromise even more severe than that of smokers. Individuals who have active autoimmune diseases such as scleroderma, lupus, or Sjogren's disease specifically affecting the face are also at a higher risk of skin flap compromise. The decision to operate on these patients must be considered carefully and might be unwise because of poor and unpredictable healing.

Any medication allergies as well as any prescription drugs or herbal supplements the patient may be taking should be reviewed before surgery. Of particular importance are medications or supplements that may prolong clotting times and thereby increase the chance of intraoperative bleeding and/or the risk of hematoma (**Table 1**). The use of such medications should be stopped at least 2 weeks before surgery, under the supervision of the patient's primary care physician. Additionally, the authors recommend a perioperative regimen of vitamin C and *Arnica Montana* to

Table 1 Medications and supplements that interfere with blood clotting	
Medication/Supplement	**Examples**
Health food/vitamin supplements	St John's wort, ginkgo biloba, vitamin E (megadoses)
Nonsteroidal anti-inflammatory drugs	Ibuprofen, indomethacin, naproxen, nabumetone
Anti-inflammatory medications	Toltetrin, dipyridamole, fenoprofen
All aspirin-containing medications	

promote healing and reduce postoperative bruising and edema.

EXAMINATION/FACIAL ANALYSIS

The examination and facial analysis is an extension of the history-taking portion of the consultation and often is performed in fluid continuity with this discussion. It is important to discuss and have the patient consider the genetic influence of the patient's current appearance as well as the gravitational effects working in concert with the hereditary loss of elasticity of the skin and changes in the underlying adipose and bony structural tissues. This consideration carefully guides the patient's understanding of what needs to be accomplished in a rhytidectomy operation to "turn back the clock," both from a conceptual and anatomical standpoint. Additionally, each patient should understand how the patient's social history has influenced the aging process. Sun exposure, in particular exposure to UVA radiation, periods of stress in the patient's life, hormonal changes, and smoking habits can contribute to the development of the sagging, aging face.

It is particularly important to point out the influence of physical habitus on the expected outcome and any favorable or unfavorable characteristics the patient may possess (**Box 1**). Although obesity is not a contraindication to rhytidectomy, it is important to explain in the preoperative discussion that results are less predictable and shorter-lived in obese individuals. In fact, patients who have a heavy "bull" neck often require a submental tuck-up within 12 to 18 months. If a patient is actively dieting or losing weight, the authors encourage the patient to postpone surgery until a stable and ideal weight has been achieved.

Once it is clear that the surgeon's ability and the patient's motivations are reciprocal, a thorough examination is performed in front of a mirror with a specific demonstration of what a facelift will do and what it will not do. This discussion includes a visual description of the proper vectors for lifting the neck and jaw line.

Patients frequently present with one of four main areas of concern relating to their midface, lower face, and neckline.

1. Neck, skin, and fat ptosis with either a double chin or banding. A patient might state specifically, "I just want my neck tightened," and in the same breath might state, "but I don't want a facelift." This statement might be true in a younger patient, who might need only submental work performed, but in most of the aging population the skin has lost its elasticity

---

Box 1
"Favorable characteristics" and "unfavorable characteristics" for facelift candidates
Favorable characteristics
Strong forward chin
Prominent cheek structure
Good facial bone structure
Fuller midface
Sharp cervicomental angle
Shallow cheek/lip grooves
Nonsmoker
Good skin tone
Few wrinkles with minimal photoaging
Unfavorable characteristics
Retrognathic or weak chin
Deep oral commissure grooves
Thin skin
Severely wrinkled and sun-damaged skin
Low hyoid with obtuse cervicomental angle
Deep cheek/lip grooves
Weak cheek bones
Deficient midface tissues
Visible submandibular glands

---

and needs to be pulled back, redraped, and trimmed. Educating the patient and alleviating the fear and misconceptions about a facelift will go a long way toward preparing the patient for surgery.

2. Increasing development of jowls with loss of definition of the submandibular jaw line and the increasing formation of the oral commissure-chin-cheek groove (the "marionette line"). The facelift procedure does an excellent job in defining the jaw line. Patients also are informed that the oral commissure groove is improved significantly, but the downward turn of the oral commissure often is not affected by facelifting. Injectable fillers are suggested if this is an area of great concern to the individual.

3. Deepening cheek/lip grooves. A conscious effort is made to point out that the cheek/lip groove is minimally effaced with most facelift techniques and the redundancy of the melolabial fold is improved only partially. Injectable fillers serve as a nice adjunctive procedure to improve this area. The patient actually might lift the mid-cheek tissues at malar eminence and lateral canthus, saying, "This is all I want,

a little tuck." Most SMAS facelift procedures do a poor job in this region. As stated, a SMAS facelift may improve the lower half of the cheek-lip groove slightly, but the effect is not universally long lasting. The midface lift is the procedure of choice for rejuvenation of this area. Facial rhytids are discussed also. These rhytids may improve somewhat following the procedure, but in many cases this improvement is only temporary and disappears as edema resolves and rebound relaxation takes effect.

4. Chin augmentation. Finally, the extent of the chin and jaw line in relationship to the cervical mental angle is evaluated, and augmentation of the mentum to achieve the best aesthetic profile is suggested in appropriate cases.

Each anatomical point discussed in front of the mirror then is reconfirmed with video imaging, which allows the patient to compare a projected result with the preoperative condition. Imaging further depicts the limitations of the operation based on the underlying physical structure and existing asymmetries.

The consultation is concluded by making sure the patient understands the expected healing times and any limitations on work or social activities. All the potential normal sequelae of facelifting surgery, as well as the potential risks and complications, are covered in detail.

TYPES OF FACELIFTS

Through many years of experience in aging face surgery, the senior author has developed a philosophical approach toward rhytidectomy that closely reflects his clinical understanding of the facial aging process. Although a variety of surgical techniques have been described through the years, the ultimate goal has remained the same: to provide a rejuvenated appearance that is both natural and long-lasting. To hold true to this goal, the facial plastic surgeon must transcend a cookbook approach to facelift surgery and, instead, base his or her approach on a dedicated effort to understand a patient's unique facial characteristics. At consultation, each patient is considered individually with respect to his or her personal concerns and fears, pre-existing facial and neck anatomy, and hairline/hairstyle. Rhytidectomy candidates can be divided into three basic categories (types I, II, or III) depending on the degree of excess submental fat, platysmal banding, overall skin thickness, and skin laxity. In the modified deep-plane extended rhytidectomy technique, a graduated approach is used for each patient to achieve the expected and desired result.

A type I facelift candidate has minimal laxity in the jowls and neck (**Fig. 1**A, B), requiring a shorter elevation and undermining of the SMAS with imbrication. Liposuction is not necessary or is minimally performed in the submental region. The difference between plication and imbrication is important. Imbrication involves elevation and redraping of the SMAS. The excess SMAS then is trimmed and generally is sutured end-to-end to the proximal (posterior) incised edge of the SMAS. The authors, however, anchor the SMAS in a bi-directional manner to a periosteum of the posterior zygoma (upper limb) and the mastoid periosteum (inferior limb). Plication, on the other hand, involves folding the SMAS upon itself by suturing it posteriorly without elevating it. The authors prefer to use the imbrication technique for most patients, because it (1) provides a more stable fixation point (the periosteum is much less subject to laxity); (2) introduces a supportive "sling effect" that repositions the lax and sagging tissues; and (3) provides a more lasting result because of the introduction of a full layer of scar to support the SMAS.

A type II facelift, which is by far the most common, requires a moderate degree of liposuction to thin the jowl and neck tissues, a moderate degree of platysma excision with plication and full undermining of the neck skin, a significant degree of SMAS undermining with imbrication, and release of the malar attachments in the midcheek (**Fig. 2**A, B).

A candidate for a type III facelift has a very heavy neck. Such patients often have a low-positioned hyoid and significant laxity of the submental skin. These patients often do not have a clear separation of the transition between the jaw line and the neck. Men usually are in this category because of their bearded, heavy, thick skin and their tendency to develop large skin wattles. Often, contouring the neck by liposuction and plication of the platysmal bands in a type III patient requires twice the time needed for a type I or II patient. The focus of the operation is creating a new defined neck angle. These patients also have deep cheek/lip grooves and melolabial folds with loss of support of the mid-cheek tissues. The SMAS flap is widely elevated, with extension nearly to the midface if possible. These patients often benefit from midface lift procedures (**Fig. 3**A, B).

SURGICAL PLANNING FOR FACELIFT

Proper incision planning and marking are crucial to achieve long-term patient satisfaction. Avoiding changes to the hairline and visible scars is critical to a successful outcome. Patients who have well-hidden scars and unchanged hairlines have

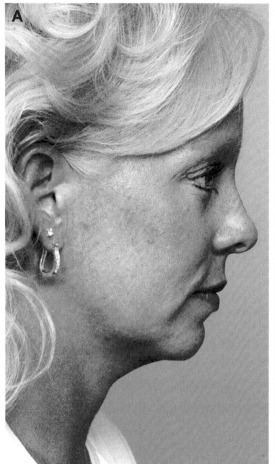 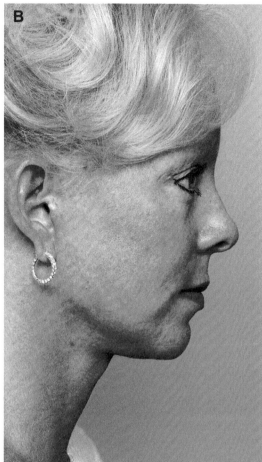

Fig. 1. (*A* Preop, *B* Postop) A type I facelift candidate.

more freedom in styling their hair, leading to greater satisfaction. Often, the surgeon who takes care in incision planning will receive referrals from hairdressers and aestheticians who recognize superior results.[5] In considering the placement of incisions, three points must be considered.

The first is maintaining the preauricular tuft of hair, including the sideburn. The location of the lower portion of the sideburn and the width at which it extends anteriorly from the insertion of the helical curvature differ in each patient. If the preauricular tuft is 1 or 2 cm below the insertion of the superior portion of the helical insertion, it may be appropriate to design an incision that curves up into the temporal hair and allows some posterior superior lifting of the hairline. The curved hairline incision rather than a straight vertical incision is required to interrupt forces of contracture, to reduce scar widening, and to avoid alopecia. As long as the hairline is not lifted higher than the superior helical insertion, there will be no significant cosmetic disturbance of the area. If the

sideburn is at the helical insertion preoperatively, an incision at the inferior border of the sideburn is required. At no time should the incision be carried anteriorly around the sideburn tuft and along the pretemporal hairline. All scars in this area will be visible and cannot be camouflaged by the fine, severely sloped hair as it exits the skin naturally in a posterior direction. All incisions should be beveled to allow hair regrowth through scars created during incision.[6]

Second, the preauricular incision starts at the helical insertion and follows the apparent curvatures of the auricle itself to the helical root. The incision continues 1 to 2 mm behind the tragus and exits at the junction of the earlobe with the face. In male patients, a pretragal incision is used to avoid lifting and placing hair-bearing skin over the tragus (**Fig. 4**).

Third, the postauricular incision must be directed up onto the posterior aspect of the auricle. The incision is placed above the sulcus so that when the ear settles posteriorly and the

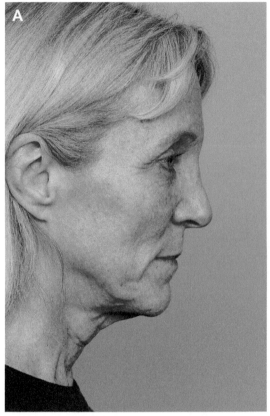 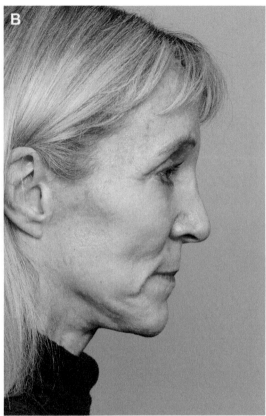

Fig. 2. (*A* Preop, *B* Postop) A type II facelift candidate.

scar heals with some contracture of the skin, the scar falls into the sulcus and does not migrate.

At the level of the helical insertion or eminence of the concha, the incisions curve gently toward the hairline. Depending on the laxity of the skin that must to be removed from the neckline, the incision is directed horizontally through the hairline (for minimal skin laxity) or down along the hairline (for greater skin laxity). When the postauricular skin is advanced posteriorly and superiorly, the posterior hairline can be approximated with no step-off or other deformity (**Fig. 5**).[7]

SURGICAL TECHNIQUE FOR FACELIFT

The beginning of the facelift operation requires treatment of the neck first, before the posterior shortening and suspension of the platysma muscle. In addition, treating the fatty tissues of the jowl, the submentum, submandibular region, and neck sets the stage for proper contouring of the neck and jaw line with treatment of the SMAS tissues. The procedure is started by making a 2- to 3-cm incision in the submental crease, followed by 0.5-cm elevation of the skin to expose the subcutaneous tissue. After hemostasis is

achieved, a small 3-mm, round liposuction cannula with three rectangular holes on one side is used to pre-elevate tunnels into the jowl in a radial, fanlike fashion from the left submandibular area completely to the submandibular area on the right. Once pre-tunneling has been accomplished, a judicious liposuction at 1 atmosphere of pressure of each jowl is performed to avoid dimpling. Symmetric and adequate liposuction can be accomplished by using the nondominant hand to palpate the jowls, then lifting the tissues and excess fat into the cannula. To avoid dimpling, care should be taken to avoid turning the holes of the cannula toward the dermis. For patients who have significant lipoptosis, a 5-mm spatula liposuction cannula can be used in addition to the 3-mm cannula in the central neck compartment. Liposuction contributes greatly to the overall initial and long-term results in facelift, with the caveat that one should err on the conservative side of fat reduction in any specific compartment. Overzealous suctioning may make the ptotic submandibular gland more visible and thus a more difficult aesthetic issue for the patient.[8]

In most types of facelift, further work is required to tighten the ptotic anterior platysma muscle and

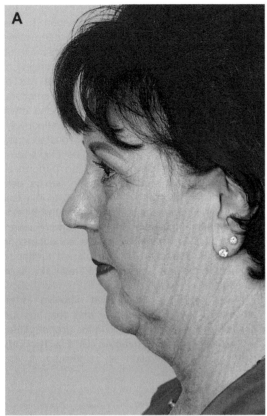

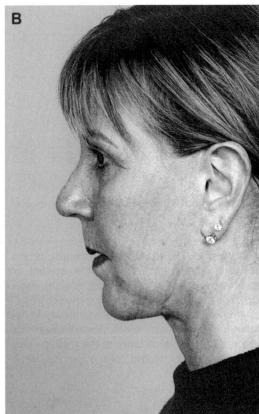

Fig. 3. (A, B) Type III facelift candidates.

to remove some subplatysmal fat in the anterior midline area. The authors favor the Kelly clamp technique for submental platysmaplasty because it provides safe, reliable results. To accomplish the Kelly clamp platysmaplasty, complete undermining of the neck skin is required. This undermining is done with Kahn beveled facelift dissection scissors. From the submental incision, the elevation is continued to the anterior part of the sterno-cleidomastoid bilaterally and across the cervicomental angle. The remaining ptotic tissue is easily visualized directly. The forceps is used to pick up the loose anterior platysmal bands as well as the subplatysmal fat that is redundant in the midline. A large, curved Kelly clamp then is used to tighten these tissues in the anterior midline. Once the anterior tissues are tightened and firm, sequential cauterization, excision, and suturing together with mattressing buried 3–0 Vicryl sutures (Ethicon, Somerville, New Jerey) is performed (**Fig. 6**). This sequential excision and suturing is done from the submental crease down to and sometimes across the cervicomental angle. Excision of digastric muscle and/or repositioning the hyoid muscle may involve more surgical

intervention than is indicated for the patient undergoing cosmetic surgery. In the patient who has a very heavy neck, 3–0 Tevdek suture is used in a figure-of-eight fashion to oversew the anterior platysmal plication. Thus, at this point a firm anterior corset has been created, setting the stage for bilateral posterior suspension and imbrication of

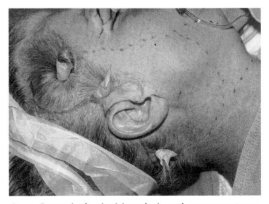

Fig. 4. Preauricular incision designed to prevent pre-tragal scarring and to protect the preauricular hair tuft.

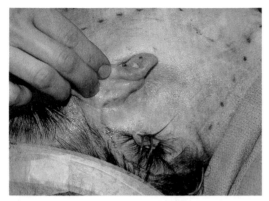

Fig. 5. Postauricular incision just above sulcus and across the hairline.

the platysma.[9] The extent of undermining of the neck skin is related directly to the amount of redundancy of skin in the neck and whether excisional plication of the platysma is required.

The neck skin is undermined completely to redrape these tissues in a posterior–superior fashion. The degree of laxity in the midface and concerns about the viability of the skin flap often dictate a lesser degree of undermining in the mid-cheek tissues and more attention to the underlying structures via the deep-plane approach. Sub-SMAS and deep-plane techniques in the midface require much less undermining of the facial skin, thereby decreasing the risk of vascular compromise, particularly in smokers. The number of seromas, hematomas, and other irregularities in this area also is reduced effectively.

After temporal, preauricular, and postauricular incisions have been fashioned and beveled appropriately, skin flap elevation can be performed. Elevation of the postauricular skin flap is performed first. Dissection begins deep to the hair follicles and superficial to the fascia of the sternocleidomastoid muscle and then turns more superficial until it is in the immediate subcutaneous plane. This dissection can be carried further to connect to the previously elevated neck skin flaps if necessary.

Using Kahn beveled facelift scissors in an advanced spread technique with the tips up assures that the dissection is in the proper plane.

Next, attention is directed to the temporal region, where elevation is performed in the

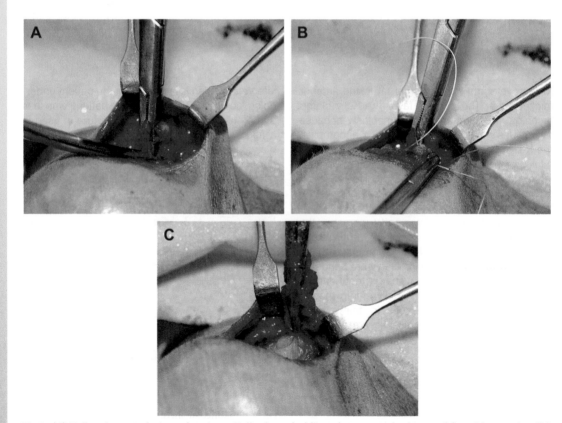

Fig. 6. (*A*) Kelley clamp technique showing a Kelly clamp holding platysma and submental fat with superior division by scissors. (*B*) Vicryl suture corset of medial platysmal edges. (*C*) Near-complete removal of contents.

subgaleal supratemporalis fascia plane all the way to the lateral orbital rim. Dissection is continued in this plane down near the upper border of the zygomatic arch. If an inferior sideburn incision has been made, a disconnected temporal incision is made to accomplish this temporal lift. Preauricular skin elevation then is begun at the level of the helical insertion and in the subcutaneous plane. Initial dissection begins beneath the hair follicles of the sideburn and then extends out in the subcutaneous plane to the lateral orbital crow's-feet region. This dissection can be done safely in the subcutaneous plane without risk of injury to the frontal branch of the facial nerve coursing just beneath this level of dissection. As long as one preserves the layer within the temporalis fascia in a subcutaneous plane, there is no risk to the frontal branch of the facial nerve from direct dissection. Elevation is continued approximately 3 to 4 cm in the preauricular region connecting down to the elevated neck and postauricular flaps.

Once hemostasis is obtained, one can visualize all the way down below the mandibular margin into the neck (**Fig. 7**). An incision then is made in the SMAS extending from the inferior border of the zygomatic arch at the malar eminence diagonally down to the level of the earlobe and continuing inferiorly 1 cm in front of the anterior border of the sternocleidomastoid. The first centimeter of SMAS elevation is performed with horizontal scissor dissection. Further elevation of the SMAS is performed by spreading the scissors in a more vertical fashion, directly visualizing tunnels and bridges as the dissection is carried anteriorly. Dissection is carried 3 to 4 cm underneath the platysma muscle. Just above the mandibular margin, dissection is continued superficial to the masseter muscle over the premasseteric fascia. The marginal mandibular nerve often is visualized easily. Dissection then is begun in the malar region

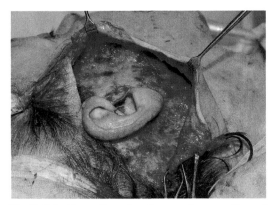

Fig. 7. Skin flap after elevation and connection of cheek and neck flaps.

just above the zygomatic buttress in the subcutaneous plane extending just inferior to the orbicularis muscle. This dissection requires the release of strong dermal attachments to the malar eminence. Some control of bleeding often is required. Elevation then is extended easily superficial to the level of the zygomaticus muscle and into the mid-cheek region if necessary. Individualization of the extent of mid-cheek SMAS undermining is important. Not all patients require full SMAS elevation of the mid-cheek, as has been reported for the standard deep-plane facelift. Once good mobilization of the jowl and malar eminence has been accomplished, a complete elevation transition from deep to superficial to the zygomaticus muscle generally is not required. Increased safety is the benefit of modifying the deep-plane technique, which leaves the zygomatic and buccal branches of the facial nerve in less danger of injury.

The other modification by which this technique differs from a standard deep-plane technique is the elevation of 4 cm of skin in addition to the SMAS, creating two separate flaps for later biplane vector suspension. At this stage, the suspension of the midface and jowl tissues is accomplished by advancing the SMAS–subcutaneous skin unit in a posterior–superior fashion. Because there are significant skin–dermal adipose–SMAS fibrous connections, the mobilization of the SMAS provides a tremendous lift and improvement of the lower and midface. In addition, the soft tissues of the midface are elevated in continuity with this compound unit. The superior triangular portion of the SMAS is advanced, and Metzenbaum scissors are used to incise the redundant preauricular portion of the SMAS. The superior slip of this SMAS is left intact and is suspended to the dense preauricular temporalis fascia at the level of the helical insertion with a deep, buried 0 Vicryl suture. Occasionally, a secondary support of one 3–0 Tevdek suture is used in a patient who has a heavy cheek. Attention then is directed toward the overlapping platysma-SMAS at the level of the earlobe. Metzenbaum scissors are used to incise this tissue so a posterior–inferior slip of platysma-SMAS can be suspended intact to the mastoid fascia with a 0 Vicryl suture (**Fig. 8**). This maneuver literally hangs the platysma from the mastoid, creating a firm corset across the midline to the opposite side.

Some redundant fatty tissue and SMAS overlapping the lower portions of the sternocleidomastoid are trimmed to avoid extra lumpiness in this area. Then, 3–0 polydioxanone sutures (Ethicon, Somerville, New Jersey) are used to reinforce the platysma–SMAS unit to the posterior mastoid-sternocleidomastoid fascia. The preauricular area

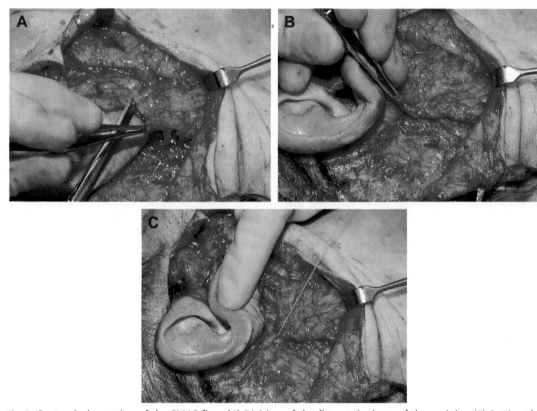

Fig. 8. Postauricular setting of the SMAS flap. (*A*) Division of the flap at the base of the earlobe. (*B*) Setting the flap in a posterior superior direction over the mastoid. (*C*) Vicryl suturing of flap into position.

also is trimmed and sutured end to end with 3–0 polydioxanone sutures to complete the SMAS imbrication. If only a small amount of jowl repositioning and posterior repositioning of the platysma muscle are required, plication of the SMAS may be the only maneuver necessary.

At this stage, the skin is easily advanced up and redraped over the auricle in a different, more posterior vector. Only 2 to 3 cm of undermined skin remain in the preauricular region. The skin from the neck is advanced to the posterior mastoid hairline region posteriorly, and then it is rotated superiorly. These three different lifting vectors achieve an effect similar to that described by Baker[7] with the triplane rhytidectomy, ensuring the re-creation and maintenance of the postauricular hairline and avoiding step-off deformity. A single suspension suture is placed in the high postauricular region. Next, the hair-bearing portions are re-approximated with staples, and the skin is sutured with 5–0 plain interlocking catgut suture. The preauricular skin is moved in a much more posterior direction (rather than superior) to avoid any undue movement of the temporal hairline.

The skin is trimmed judiciously in the preauricular area, ensuring that the earlobe is cradled in a superior fashion to avoid a satyr's ear deformity and a migrating scar in this region.

The tragal flap is designed to be extremely redundant, and it is sutured in a running interlocking fashion with a 5–0 plain catgut suture. No tension is left on the tragal skin, and the skin is thinned judiciously to avoid overthinning and loss of viability. The closure in the temporal hair-bearing portion of the skin is performed by incrementally excising the redundancy and placing one buried 3–0 Vicryl suture that holds the galeal suspension to the temporalis fascia. The scalp then is approximated with interrupted staples. Just before the conclusion of the closure, a drain is placed into the neck portion of the wound on either side. This precaution reduces the rates of hematomas and seromas significantly. A permanent 6–0 nylon suture is placed at the earlobe and is left in place for 10 days. The remainder of the skin closure is performed with catgut sutures (which either dissolve or are removed at 1 week). Placement of the drain also reduces the need for any kind of compressive dressing, but a light

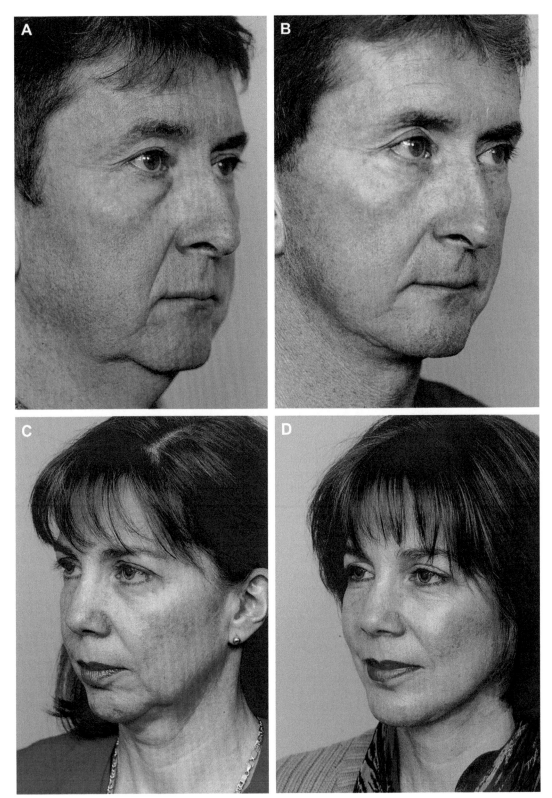

Fig. 9. (*A*, *C*, *E*) Preoperative and (*B*, *D*, *F*) postoperative photographs of three patients showing natural-looking, long-lasting results.

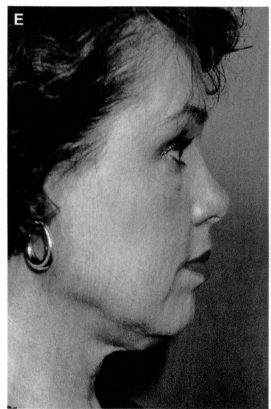

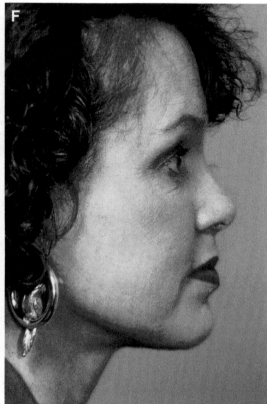

Fig. 9. (*continued*)

compression dressing using an abdominal dressing/combined dressing and elastic chin strap is used for patient and family convenience. Mild compression is used in the preauricular area to prevent any fluid collection in this region.[10] Significant compression dressings used in the past without suction drainage increased the incidence of problems with skin viability.

Pressure dressings can create poor venous outflow and skin necrosis, which can occur from venous congestion even when arterial vascular perfusion is adequate. Slow venous flow within the flap increases the chance of infection, further inflaming the flap and creating loss of perfusion and, ultimately, potential loss of viability.[11]

After the appropriate initial follow-up to ensure proper healing, all patients are followed for at least 1 year, when postoperative results are accessed and photographs are taken. Most patients continue to return for follow-up for years to monitor the lasting results of their facelifts (**Fig. 9**).

COMPLICATIONS IN FACELIFT
Hematoma

Hematoma is the most common complication following rhytidectomy; in the senior author's experience, it occurs approximately 1% to 2% of the time. The incidence in the literature varies from 2% to 15%.[10] In the senior author's experience, seromas occur in 2% of patients. The low occurrence of seromas is attributed to the placement of bulb suction drains.

Infection

Infection can occur in approximately 4% to 5% of patients during cephalosporin prophylaxis. Any signs of unilateral erythema in the pre- or postauricular regions, increasing pain, or delayed wound healing at the edges are treated with aggressive antibiotic coverage to target *Pseudomonas* and other gram-negative bacilli. Abscesses occur in less than 0.2% of patients and require immediate drainage and broad-spectrum antibiotic coverage.

Skin Necrosis

Skin necrosis can be a deforming complication that is seen more commonly in smokers. In fact, the risk of skin flap death is 12% higher in smokers than in nonsmokers.[11]

Facial Nerve Injury

Although it has been reported that facial nerve injury can occur in 0.5% to 6.0% of all patients undergoing facelift, it never should occur, even with the deep-plane techniques available today.[12] In nearly 2000 patients, the only facial nerve occurrences were two cases of temporal frontal branch paresis, caused by stretching the nerve while elevating the temporal portion of the skin flap. Both these injuries resolved within 2 to 4 months. With meticulous dissection techniques in the midface region, the use of this modified SMAS elevation should prevent any injury to the facial nerve.

SUMMARY

A facial plastic surgeon has an obligation to deliver confidently the result that one promises. It also is important that one like the result one delivers. Through 26 years of experience performing rhytidectomy, the senior author has come to rely on a graduated approach toward rhytidectomy that consistently has afforded the desired natural-looking result. This success relies on accurate patient analysis.

As a surgeon gains experience, further improvements can be gained with more aggressive surgery, but complications begin to occur when more aggressive measures are undertaken. Therefore, the ideal technique is one that maximizes rejuvenation while minimizing adverse effects. The senior author has found that the aggressive techniques in the region of the neck have improved dramatically the overall initial and long-term results for the neck portion of the rhytidectomy. More aggressive treatment of the midface during the modified deep-plane rhytidectomy does not necessarily improve the overall long-term results, however, and can increase the complication rate. Adjunctive procedures (ie, skin resurfacing, injectable fillers, botulinum toxin type A injections) and other surgical procedures (ie, midface lift, chin implantation) can be used to complement the results of rhytidectomy.

REFERENCES

1. Foment S. The surgery of injury and plastic repair. Baltimore (MD): Williams & Wilkins; 1939.
2. Skoog T. Plastic surgery: the aging face. In: Skoog T, editor. Plastic surgery: new methods and refinements. Philadelphia: WB Saunders; 1974. p. 300–30.
3. Mitz V, Peyronie M. The superficial musculo-aponeurotic system (SMAS) in the parotid and cheek area. Plast Reconstr Surg 1990;86:53–61.
4. Lemmon ML, Hamra ST. Skoog rhytidectomy: a five-year experience with 577 patients. Plast Reconstr Surg 1980;65:283–97.
5. Hamra ST. The deep plane rhytidectomy. Plast Reconstr Surg 1990;86:53–61.
6. Kamer FM. One hundred consecutive deep plane face lifts. Arch Otolaryngol Head Neck Surg 1996; 122:17–22.
7. Baker SR. Tri-plane rhytidectomy. Arch Otolaryngol Head Neck Surg 1997;123:1167–72.
8. Ramirez OM. The subperiosteal rhytidectomy: the third generation facelift. Ann Plast Surg 1992;28: 218–32.
9. Koch BB, Perkins SW. Simultaneous rhytidectomy and full-face carbon dioxide laser resurfacing: a case series and meta-analysis. Arch Facial Plast Surg 2002;4:227–33.
10. Perkins SW, Williams JD, MacDonald K, et al. Prevention of seromas and hematomas following facelift surgery with the use of postoperative vacuum drains. Arch Otolaryngol Head Neck Surg 1997;123:743–5.
11. Straith RE, Raju D, Hipps C. The study of hematomas in 500 consecutive face lifts. Plast Reconstr Surg 1977;59:694–8.
12. Castanares S. Facial nerve paralyses coincident with or subsequent to rhytidectomy. Plast Reconstr Surg 1974;54:637–43.

Rejuvenation of the Aging Neck: Current Principles, Techniques, and Newer Modifications

David A. Caplin, MD[a],*, Chad A. Perlyn, MD, PhD[b]

KEYWORDS

- Neck • Neck-lift • Rhytidectomy • Platysmaplasty
- Cervicomental angle • Facial rejuvenation

Aesthetic improvement of the neck and cervicomental (CM) angle remains one of the most challenging aspects of surgical facial rejuvenation. Individuals may become dissatisfied with the appearance of their neck because of changes in skin quality, submental fat, and muscle tone or position related to aging, weight gain, weight loss, sun damage, and other causes. To achieve the patient's desired result, surgeons use various techniques, either in isolation or in combination. Careful preoperative evaluation of the patient's anatomy dictates the most appropriate procedure, ranging from traditional or laser-assisted lipolysis (LAL) to sub-superficial muscular aponeurotic system (sub-SMAS) rhytidectomy with an extended platysmaplasty. This article reviews the techniques that are available and the decision-making process used in choosing the most appropriate technique for each patient.

The key question for the surgeon is "What defines an aesthetically pleasing neck?" When presenting for evaluation, patients often pull and pinch their neck to attempt to demonstrate their neck of earlier years. Numerous studies have shown that a youthful-appearing neck has an acute CM angle (105° to 120°), a distinct inferior mandibular border, and a visible anterior border of the sternocleidomastoid

muscle.[1,2] A noticeable thyroid cartilage and subthyroid depression also contribute to the attractiveness of the neck.[1] To characterize the aging process in the neck and lower face, several classification schemes have been developed. The Dedo system is based on anatomic layers[3]:

- Class I describes a youthful neck with a well-defined CM angle, excellent platysmal tone, and no submental fat.
- A class II neck presents with simple skin laxity without submental fat or loss of platysmal tone.
- Class III necks have accumulation of submental fat.
- Class IV describes platysmal banding.
- Class V and VI necks are based on bony structure, with retrognathic patients having class V necks and those with low hyoid bones having class VI neck.

Baker has developed a similar classification that defines four subtypes of patients seeking jowl and neck rejuvenation[4]:

- Type I patients have slight cervical skin laxity with submental fat and early jowls.
- Type II patients have moderate cervical skin laxity, moderate jowls and submental fat.

An educational grant for the artwork presented in this article was provided by Cynosure and Dr Caplin is a Cynosure Clinical Consultant.
[a] Division of Parkcrest Plastic Surgery, University of Washington, 845 N. New Ballas Court, Suite # 300, St Louis, MO 63141, USA
[b] Florida International University, College of Medicine, 11200 SW, 8th Street, HLS II 693, Miami, FL 33199, USA
* Corresponding author.
E-mail address: Gfts27@aol.com (D.A. Caplin).

Facial Plast Surg Clin N Am 17 (2009) 589–601
doi:10.1016/j.fsc.2009.07.001
1064-7406/09/$ – see front matter © 2009 Elsevier Inc. All rights reserved.

- Type III patients have moderate cervical skin laxity, but with significant jowling and active platysmal banding.
- Type IV patients have loose, redundant cervical skin and folds below the cricoid, significant jowls, and active platysmal bands.[4]

The authors prefer to use the Baker scale for patient evaluation, and most commonly encounter individuals with type II and III necks. This article focuses on these groups of patients.

Many methods have been described for rejuvenating an aging neck and each technique is a variation on a larger theme. These include skin tightening/excision procedures, platysmal tightening, digastric modification, suspension sutures, fat removal, and chemodenervation (botulinum toxin type A). When a patient is interested in undergoing rejuvenation of the neck, it is important to analyze his or her anatomic findings to best define the surgical and nonsurgical options for reconstruction. This article presents a combination of established techniques that can be used as part of a cervicofacial rhytidectomy or in cases of isolated neck rejuvenation. The aged neck can be successfully recontoured using the proper sequence of lipectomy, skin undermining, muscle plication, and, if needed, suspension sutures. In addition, adjuvant techniques such as fat grafting, stem-cell rich autologous fibrin glue, and injection of botulinum toxin A can improve surgical results and patient satisfaction.

RELEVANT ANATOMY

One should not attempt to rejuvenate an aged neck without a thorough understanding of normal neck anatomy and the relationships of critical structures to cervicomental aesthetics.[2,5,6] The surface landmarks of the neck begin at the pericraniocervical line and end at the level of the clavicle. Between the break point of the vertical portion of the neck and the transverse portion of the submandibular region is the CM angle,[5] which corresponds to the position of the hyoid bone relative to the mandible. The hyoid bone typically lies at the level of the third cervical vertebrae. A low hyoid bone or a recessed mandible will alter the point of transition from the vertical plane to the transverse and affect the CM angle. Below the hyoid bone is the thyroid cartilage and the prominent laryngeal prominence (Adam's apple). This prominence is visible in men, but is not normally apparent in women.

Below the skin of the neck, with its blood supply from the transverse cervical branch of the subclavian artery and the superior thyroid artery, is a layer of subcutaneous fat, the thickness of which varies with age and weight. Care must be taken when removing subcutaneous cervical fat to avoid masculinization, which can be caused by visualization of the thyroid cartilage. Interposed between the subcutaneous fat and the deep structures of the neck is the platysma muscle, which attaches to the cervicopectoral fascia inferiorly and to the depressor anguli oris, risorius, and mentalis muscles superiorly. It follows a course from superomedial to inferolateral bilaterally, with a variable amount of decussation in the midline. With aging, the platysma is pulled laterally, resulting in splaying of the medial fibers and the development of dynamic platysmal bands, which are often exacerbated with contraction of the platysma. In addition, the decussation of the platysma and loss of muscle tone allow for herniation of subplatysmal fat. When fat is excised from this area, the bilateral anterior jugular veins must be avoided or cauterized to prevent excessive bleeding during the dissection.

Deep to the platysma lie the major neurovascular structures of the neck. The marginal mandibular and cervical branches of the facial nerve are at risk of injury during neck rejuvenation. The marginal mandibular nerve runs toward the mandibular angle in a subplatysmal plane before turning across the body of the mandible to supply the muscles of the lower lip and chin. In approximately 40% of individuals, the marginal mandibular branch passes 1.2 to 1.3 cm below the body of the mandible.[7] The danger zone for injuring the marginal mandibular branch encompasses laterally the angle of the mandible, medially to the oral commissure, a line 2 cm below and parallel to the mandibular border caudally, and a line 1 cm above and parallel to the inferior border of the mandible cephalically.[8] The cervical branch runs anteroinferiorly under the platysma to supply the platysma. The external jugular vein is also encountered deep to the platysma during lateral dissection. It is separated from the sternocleidomastoid muscle by the investing layer of the deep cervical fascia. Its upper half runs parallel to the greater auricular nerve. The greater auricular nerve crosses the sternocleidomastoid muscle 6.0 to 6.5 cm inferior to the external auditory meatus, where it divides into its auricular, mastoid, and facial branches.[2,9]

Other structures of relevance that are deep to the plane of the platysma are the anterior bellies of the digastric muscles and the submandibular glands. The superior attachment of the anterior belly of the digastric is to the medial surface of the parasymphyseal portion of the mandible bilaterally. It courses inferolaterally to attach to the lesser cornu of the hyoid bone by way of an aponeurosis. The position of this muscle and its action in elevating the hyoid may contribute to the appearance of the CM angle. Lying superior to the digastric muscles are the submandibular glands, which are divided into superficial and deep lobes, separated by the mylohyoid muscles. Ptotic submandibular glands may appear as prominent bulges and give the appearance of neck fullness. When considering surgery in a patient with ptotic glands, it is important to note the altered relationship between the gland and the marginal mandibular branches, as the nerve branches are pushed anterosuperiorly from their normal anatomic position.[2]

INDICATIONS FOR NECK REJUVENATION

Table 1 outlines the common anatomic findings and the authors' approach to restoring the anatomy to a more youthful state and rejuvenating the neck. Each of the procedures is discussed below, with the primary focus on Baker type II and III necks. In these patients, many of the techniques are used in sequence. For patients with less aged necks, the authors frequently address isolated components to meet the patients' needs and aesthetic goals (see **Table 1**). As in all aesthetic surgery cases, the best results are achieved when the appropriate procedure is applied to the appropriate patient.

The ideal candidate for an isolated extended platysmaplasty with suspension suture has a poorly defined CM angle, skin of moderate thickness with a defined layer of supraplatysmal fat, no evidence of significant midfacial descent, and no significant jowl formation. The technique described does not achieve the same result as a traditional cervicofacial rhytidectomy because it is only designed to address the neck. However, the authors routinely incorporate portions of the technique when performing face-lifting procedures; many patients who request rejuvenation, but prefer to avoid a face-lift, find this procedure appealing. The limited incisions and undermining lead to a shorter recovery period than with a cervicofacial rhytidectomy and there is no scar in the preauricular area and no swelling or ecchymosis of the midface. Male patients often prefer this procedure, as it avoids the problems with shifting of hair-bearing areas that can be associated with preauricular scars. The male patient also has thicker skin, which can produce less satisfying results with a traditional face-lift technique unless it addresses each component of the aged neck.

In individuals with thin or excessively sun-damaged skin, a loss of dermal elasticity limits the ability of the skin to conform to the restored CM angle and the result may be less than optimal.

Table 1
Options for rejuvenation of the neck and improvement of the CM angle based on anatomic changes noted on physical examination. These procedures are frequently performed synchronously to optimize aesthetic outcome

Skin Excess	Subcutaneous Fat	Subplatysmal Fat	Low Hyoid	Platysmal Bands	Recessive Chin
Direct excision or Lower face-lift with or without platysmal tightening or Extended platysmaplasty with suspension suture	SAL or Laser-assisted liposuction or Judicious direct excision	Direct excision of subplatysmal fat with platysmal tightening Add digastric muscle plication and/or reduction if indicated	Suspension suture	Platysmal plication with anterior back-cut of platysmal muscle Botulinum toxin A treatment of platysmal bands (nonsurgical)	Osseous or alloplastic genioplasty or Chin augmentation using fat grafting or Orthognathic surgery if indicated

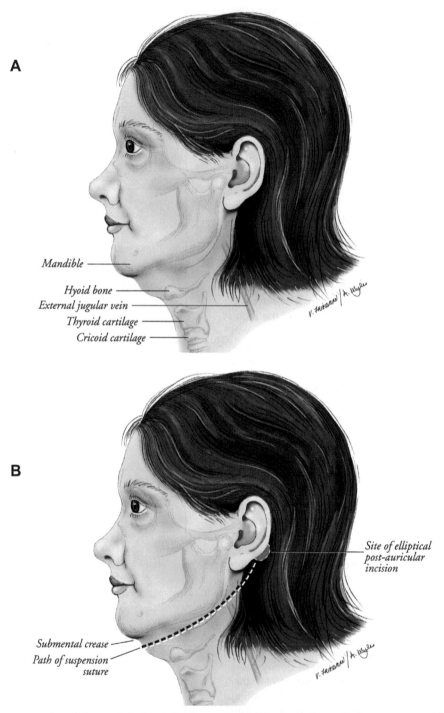

Mandible
Hyoid bone
External jugular vein
Thyroid cartilage
Cricoid cartilage

Site of elliptical
post-auricular
incision

Submental crease
Path of suspension
suture

Fig. 1. Suture suspension platysmaplasty for neck rejuvenation. (*A*) Preoperative patient appearance with submental fullness and an obtuse cervicomental angle. (*B*) Proposed path of suspension suture; note the site of a small elliptical skin incision that is performed when the procedure is not part of a rhytidectomy with a postauricular incision. (*C*) Interlocking sutures are placed in the submental region and a small liposuction cannula is passed along the proposed path of the suspension suture; the free ends of one of the sutures are placed into the cannula. (*D*) The cannula is withdrawn, dragging the sutures out behind the ear; this is repeated on the opposite side. (*E*) Tension is adjusted on the sutures until the desired appearance of the cervicomental angle is achieved. (*F*) The ends of the suture are passed into a free needle and the suture is secured to the deep mastoid fascia and tied; this is repeated on the opposite side. Note the change in the CM angle between (*A*) and (*F*).

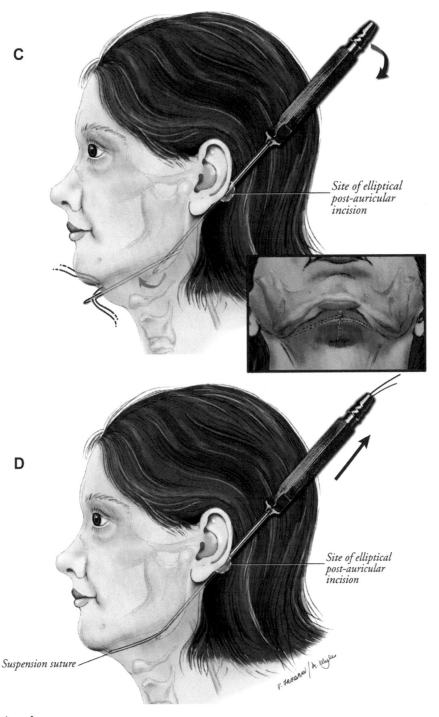

C

Site of elliptical post-auricular incision

D

Site of elliptical post-auricular incision

Suspension suture

V. FRIEDMAN / A. Kaylee

Fig. 1. (*continued*)

Patients with dramatically obese necks are also poor candidates for the procedure. In these patients, we often recommend a combination of lifestyle modification, diet, and cervical and submental liposuction. Once the neck is "deflated," the CM angle can be restored and excess skin removed.

TECHNIQUE FOR EXTENDED PLATYSMAPLASTY WITH SUSPENSION SUTURE

All markings are made with the patient in an upright position before surgery. Landmarks such as the sternocleidomastoid muscles, external

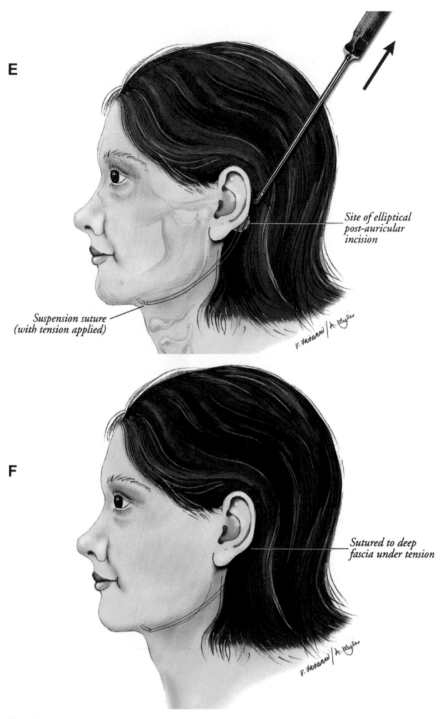

E

Site of elliptical post-auricular incision

Suspension suture (with tension applied)

F

Sutured to deep fascia under tension

Fig. 1. (*continued*)

jugular veins, platysmal bands, jowls, mastoid tip, and mandibular border are clearly marked with a surgical marking pen. The sites of the submental and postauricular incisions (elliptical skin excision), the position of the new CM angle, and the intended submandibular path of the suspension suture are also marked. After induction of general endotracheal anesthesia, approximately 15 mL of blood are drawn from an upper extremity for fabrication of the autologous fibrin glue preparation.

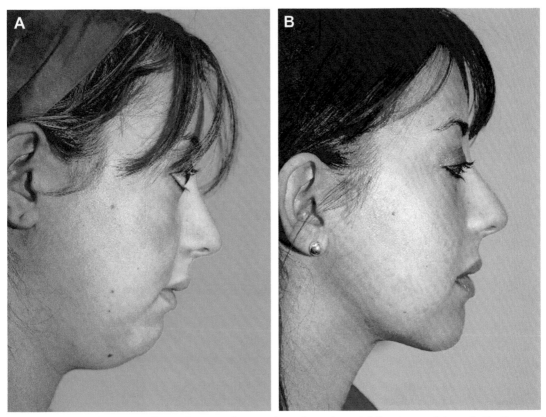

Fig. 2. A 28-year-old patient who underwent direct and suction submental lipectomy, platysmal plication, and suspension suture to improve her CM angle. Fat grafting to her chin was also performed. (*A*) Preoperative appearance. (*B*) 2-year postoperative appearance.

Although the operation may be performed under monitored anesthesia care with local anesthesia, general anesthesia has been preferred in most cases. The neck and postauricular regions are infiltrated with 0.25% lidocaine with 1:400,000 epinephrine for local hemostasis using a 25-gauge spinal needle. The sites of the submental and postauricular incisions are injected with a 27-gauge needle. The patient's neck and face are prepared using a mixture of povidone-iodine (Betadine) and alcohol, and the face, neck, and endotracheal tube are subsequently draped. The endotracheal tube is not taped to facilitate movement during surgery.

The procedure is started with a curvilinear incision within or just posterior to the first submental crease. The lateral margins of the incision may be directed posteriorly away from the mandibular border to minimize visibility of the scar. The incision length varies according to the particular situation but can be as long as 4 to 5 cm. A 3-mm spatulated liposuction cannula, or a 2-mm round cannula, is used for preplatysmal liposuction, undermining the skin flap to the level of the thyroid

notch inferiorly and as far as the external jugular veins laterally. Invariably, a perforating vein is found in the supraplatysmal plane just lateral to the lesser cornu of the hyoid bone. Face-lift scissors are then used to complete the flap elevation. In certain cases, direct excision of preplatysmal fat is warranted. A variable pocket of subplatysmal fat overlies the anterior belly of the digastric muscles, which may be partially or completely excised to optimize contour. This fat pad typically contains several vessels that bleed vigorously if not addressed with a bipolar cautery.

If necessary a variable amount of subplatysmal fat is resected and the medial edges of the anterior bellies of the digastric muscles may be exposed and sutured together using buried interrupted 4-0 braided polyester (Ethibond) sutures to even out the contour and fill the depression that may be caused by the fat removal. The digastric plication is begun at the mentum and continued as far posteriorly as possible using between three and five sutures. Hypertrophic digastric muscles can be reduced by "shaving down" the muscle belly with face-lift scissors. After performing this

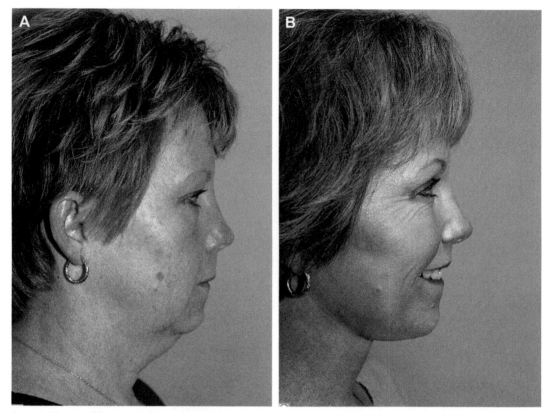

Fig. 3. A 53-year-old patient who underwent direct and suction submental lipectomy, platysmal plication, suspension suture, and rhytidectomy to improve her cervicomental angle, descent of facial soft-tissue, and jowling. (*A*) Preoperative appearance. (*B*) 2-Year postoperative appearance.

maneuver, the medial edges of the platysmal muscle are sutured using buried, interrupted 4-0 braided polyester (Ethibond) sutures. The redundant medial edges of the platysmal muscle may be excised or invaginated with the platysma sutures. During plication of the platysma, the medial edges of the muscle are back-cut transversely for 1 to 2 cm at the predetermined level of the CM angle immediately inferior to the lowest midline platysmal plication suture.

At the level of the new CM angle, a 2-0 braided polyester (Mersilene) horizontal mattress suture is placed across the previously approximated edges of the platysma muscles from right to left. This suture is interlocked with a second horizontal mattress suture (or a vertical mattress suture) from left to right in the fashion described by Giampapa (**Fig. 1**).[10] The needles are removed from the sutures and both suture ends are brought out through the submental incision and covered with a moist lap pad. When performed as an isolated neck-lift, an ellipse of skin oriented parallel to the postauricular crease is excised in the mastoid region to access the mastoid periosteum. A

2.0-mm or 2.4-mm Mercedes tip liposuction cannula is tunneled in a subcutaneous preplatysmal plane (along the previously marked submandibular line), entering the post-auricular incision and exiting the submental incision. Care is taken to avoid tunneling in a subplatysmal plane, which could cause marginal mandibular nerve injury or injury to the facial vessels. The ends of the left suture are placed through the orifice of the liposuction cannula resting in the left side of the submental incision. The cannula is then withdrawn through the subcutaneous tunnel and out of the left postauricular incision. The suture is drawn from the submental to the postauricular incision. A French-eye needle is used to secure the suture to the mastoid periosteum. Before tying the suture, an effort is made to ensure that the suture lies within the intended tunnel and does not ride up over the angle of the mandible. When the passing cannula is first introduced through the postauricular incision it allows the surgeon to preview the anticipated line-of-pull of the suspension suture as the contour of the cannula is palpable and visible through the skin. If the suture sits higher

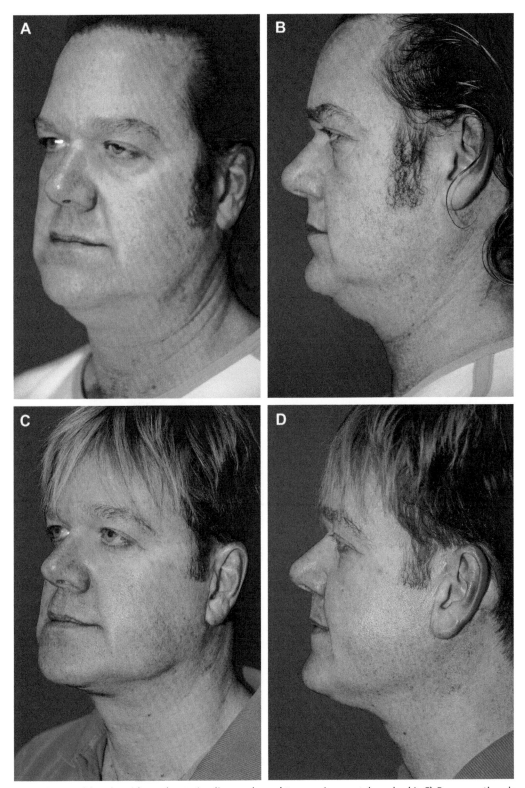

Fig. 4. A 47 year old male with moderate jowling and an obtuse cericomental angle. (*A*, *B*) Pre-operative views. (*C*, *D*) 3 months after a rhytidectomy, direct and suction submental lipectomy, plastymaplasty, suspension suture with transconjunctival lower lid blepharoplasty.

along the line of the mandible than intended, the neck will have an unnatural "creased" appearance at the angle of the mandible. If the suture is too low, a hanging submental pouch will result. When necessary the suture may be repositioned by pulling it back out through the submental incision and, once again, using the passing cannula to create a new tunnel. The suture is tied on the left with the patient's face turned toward the right. The procedure is repeated in a similar fashion on the contralateral side.

Before closure, the wound is copiously irrigated with saline. The deep portion of the postauricular incision is closed in two layers with 4-0 polygalactin sutures to ensure that the Mersilene knot does not "spit." The skin is closed with 6-0 nylon sutures. After wound irrigation and hemostasis, several milliliters of the autologous fibrin glue are squirted into the submental wound. The redundant submental skin, if any, is trimmed conservatively from the posterior edge of the submental incision. A small round drain is placed in the depths of the area of submental undermining and brought out through

an inferolateral stab incision in a neck crease and the skin margins are approximated with buried interrupted 5-0 polygalactin dermal sutures and a running subcuticular 4-0 Prolene suture. The incisions are covered with antibiotic ointment and the submental area is supported with a pad of soft foam material or roll-cotton held in place with a gauze roll and a Velcro chin-strap applied without tension. Patients are instructed to wear the compression dressing as much as possible for the first 4 to 5 days and then to wear the chin-strap at night for up to an additional 7 to 10 days. Examples of patients treated with this technique are shown in **Figs. 2–5.**

ADJUVANT TECHNIQUES FOR NECK REJUVENATION

The authors routinely use combinations of techniques when treating patients with aging necks. Descriptions of some of these techniques follow; they may be used as stand-alone treatments for the aging neck or in combination with more

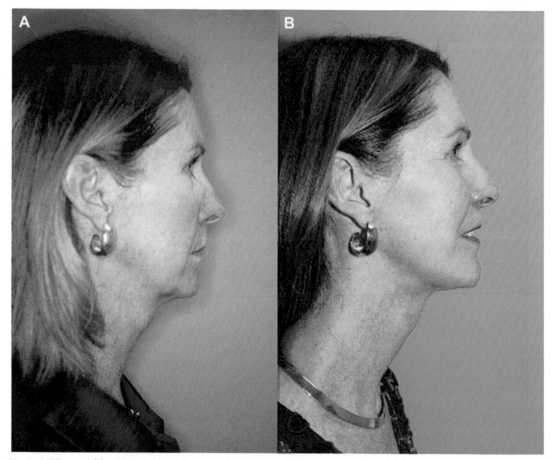

Fig. 5. A 56-year-old patient who underwent direct and suction submental lipectomy, platysmal plication, suspension suture, and rhytidectomy. (*A*) Preoperative appearance. (*B*) 2-Year postoperative appearance.

extensive procedures such as face-lifts or isolated neck-lifts.

LAL

LAL is a technique approved by the US Food and Drug Administration (FDA). The authors use a 1064-nm neodymium:yttrium aluminum garnet (Nd:YAG) laser with or without a 1320-nm component and wattage ranging from 6 W to 18 W.[11,12] This technique is effective in patients with moderate-to-full amounts of supraplatysmal fat and good skin tone. The authors have used the laser to treat subcutaneous submental fat and routinely perform the procedure under local anesthesia, although it may be combined with isolated neck-lifts or face-lifting techniques. The technique differs from conventional submental liposuction in several ways. After infiltration of the preplatysmal fat layer with tumescent solution, a 1-mm hollow cannula containing a 600-μm Nd:YAG fiber is introduced into the neck through a 2-mm stab incision in the submental crease. An additional stab incision may be made at the lower end of the nasolabial fold if the jowls are to be treated as well. The laser fiber is passed through the supraplatysmal fat, liquefying the adipose cells, and providing a hemostatic effect because of the wavelength absorption by hemoglobin. Once the supraplatysmal fat has been liquefied, secondary passes with the laser are often made along the underside of the dermis, such that the red glow of the aiming beam can be seen through the skin. This provides sufficient heat to the deep dermis to cause controlled thermal damage, inducing collagen remodeling and thermal stimulation of dermal fibroblasts. This leads to improvement in skin tone. A syringe aspiration device is then used to gently remove the liquefied fat through a 2-mm aspiration cannula. The amount of manual effort required to remove the aspirate is less than with traditional suction-assisted liposuction (SAL). This leads to less patient discomfort, less postoperative ecchymosis, and in the authors' experience, improved tolerance of the procedure when performed under local anesthesia alone. While the amount of skin tightening that occurs compared with SAL is controversial, the authors have found that the use of LAL alone has led to high levels of patient satisfaction regarding fat volume and skin tone and skin re-draping (**Fig. 6**). Recent evaluation of our results demonstrated that high levels of satisfaction with the procedure in the neck encouraged patients to have LAL on other areas of the body (unpublished data).

FAT GRAFTING

The transfer of small particles of fat from an abdominal or trunk donor site to the face for volume enhancement and rejuvenation is well described.[13–15] The authors frequently employ this technique as an adjuvant to isolated neck-lifts or when performing a cervicofacial rhytidectomy. While much of the neck-lift procedure is focused on removal of fat (preplatysmal liposuction, excision of subplatysmal fat), certain areas of the lower face will benefit from the addition of fat. One area where we sometimes employ fat grafting is the "pre-jowl" area. As the jowl descends, a depression can occur between the jowl and chin below the marionette line. Filling this depression with fat will smooth the junction between the mental area and cheek and improve the appearance of jowling and lower-face laxity. We have also treated numerous patients with small chins by performing a non-osseous autologous chin augmentation with structural fat grafting. In these patients, a small or receding chin can further contribute to a poorly defined neckline. Although many of these patients would benefit from a traditional chin augmentation, certain individuals do not want the additional recovery time of an osseous genioplasty or the problems caused by alloplastic implants. For these patients we recommend using fat to augment the chin enough to improve the lateral profile without over-augmenting the chin such that definition is lost and ptosis of the transplanted fat occurs. Extra graft material is also frequently used to fill in tear-troughs, nasolabial folds, hollow areas in the mid cheek, and "scalloping" along the lower edge of the mandible.

BOTULINUM TOXIN TYPE A

Chemodenervation of the platysma muscle using botulinum toxin type A (Botox, Allergan Irvine, CA) can reduce the appearance of prominent bands.[16,17] In patients who do not wish to undergo a more invasive rejuvenation procedure, this can be done in combination with other fillers in the upper face. Care should be taken to avoid large doses of botulinum toxin type A to the platysma in a single session because this may inadvertently affect the strap muscles of the neck. The authors have found botulinum toxin A to be beneficial in patients who present for revisional surgery of an "inverted V" deformity after a neck-lift or face-lift that did not properly address the platysmal bands. This occurs when the platysma is plicated tightly to the level of the hyoid bone, drawing the cephalic edges together, but no back-cut of the anterior platysma has been performed to transect the

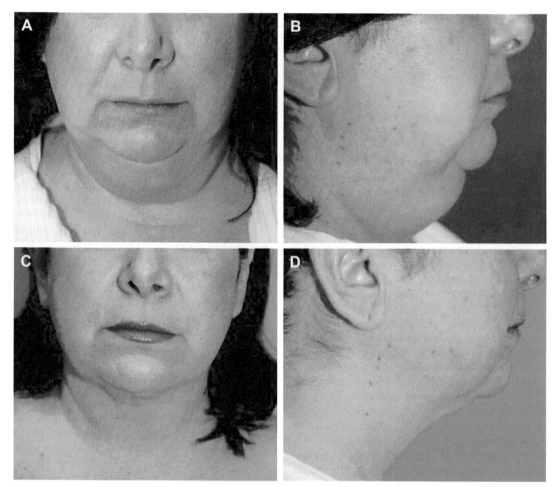

Fig. 6. A 53-year-old woman who was dissatisfied with the fullness of her neck. She was treated with LAL. (*A, B*) Preoperative views. (*C, D*) Appearance 4 months postprocedure.

bands below the level of plication. The cephalic portions of the bands are corrected, but the caudal ends may be accentuated, giving the neck an inverted V appearance. Injection of the prominent bands below the hyoid with botulinum toxin type A frequently improves this deformity without need for revision neck surgery.

SUMMARY

Rejuvenation of the neck remains a challenging procedure. Surgical treatment of the aging neck should be approached according to each patient's anatomy and aesthetic concerns. For patients with moderate cervical skin laxity, significant jowling, and active platysmal banding, the authors have found the technique described in this article to be successful. The sequence of procedures can be performed in isolation or as part of a conventional face-lift SMAS technique. In addition, portions of the technique can be selected to treat those patients who may not require so extensive a procedure. The addition of adjuvant techniques, either as part of the primary procedure, or used during revisions, has provided new tools to improve outcomes and patient satisfaction.

ACKNOWLEDGMENTS

The authors acknowledge Dr. Stephen Prendiville for his contributions to an earlier version of this manuscript, "Modifications in rejuvenation of the aging neck," published in Facial Plastic Surgery Clinics, 2002.

REFERENCES

1. Ellenbogen R, Karlin JV. Visual criteria for success in restoring the youthful neck. Plast Reconstr Surg 1980;66(6):826–37.

2. Ramírez OM. Advanced considerations determining procedure selection in cervicoplasty. Part one: anatomy and aesthetics. Clin Plast Surg 2008;35(4):679–90.

3. Dedo D. A preoperative classification of the neck for cervicofacial rhytidectomy. Laryngoscope 1984;90:1980.

4. Baker DC. Lateral SMASectomy, plication and short scar facelifts: indications and techniques. Clin Plast Surg 2008;35(4):533–50.

5. Caplin DA, Prendiville S. Modifications in rejuvenation of the aging neck. Facial Plast Surg Clin North Am 2002;10(1):77–86.

6. Prendiville S, Kokoska MS, Hollenbeak CS, et al. A comparative study of surgical techniques on the cervicomental angle in human cadavers. Arch Facial Plast Surg 2002;4:236–42.

7. Woltmann M, Faveri R, Sgrott EA. Anatomosurgical study of the marginal mandibular branch of the facial nerve for submandibular surgical approach. Braz Dent J 2006;17(1):71–4.

8. Owsley JQ, Agarwal CA. Safely navigating around the facial nerve in three dimensions. Clin Plast Surg 2008;35(4):469–77, v.

9. Alberti PW. The greater auricular nerve. Donor for facial nerve grafts: a note on its topographical anatomy. Arch Otolaryngol 1962;76:422.

10. Giampapa V, Bitzos I, Ramirez O, et al. Suture suspension platysmaplasty for neck rejuvenation revisited: technical fine points for improving outcomes. Aesthetic Plast Surg 2005;29:341–50.

11. Kim KH, Geronemus RG. Laser lipolysis using a novel 1,064 nm Nd:YAG Laser. Dermatol Surg 2006;32:241–8.

12. Goldman A. Submental Nd:Yag laser-assisted liposuction. Lasers Surg Med 2006;38:181–4.

13. Donofrio LM. Techniques in facial fat grafting. Aesthet Surg J 2008;8:681–7.

14. Locke MB. de Chala in TM. Current practice in autologous fat transplantation: suggested clinical guidelines based on a review of recent literature. Ann Plast Surg 2008;60:98–102.

15. Bucky LP, Kanchwala SK. The role of autologous fat and alternative fillers in the aging face. Plast Reconstr Surg 2007;120(Suppl 6):89S–97S.

16. Matarasso A, Matarasso SL, Brandt FS, et al. Botulinum A exotoxin for the management of platysma bands. Plast Reconstr Surg 1999;103: 645–52.

17. Brandt FS, Boker A. Botulinum toxin for the treatment of neck lines and neck bands. Dermatol Clin 2004; 22:159–66.

Surgical Treatment of the Heavy Face and Neck

Jeffrey H. Wachholz, MD[a,b],*

KEYWORDS

- Heavy neck • Facelift • Rhytidectomy
- Submental • Platysma • SMAS

Diagnosis drives treatment. We have all heard this said in various forms by mentors and respected teachers. Surgical management of the heavy neck and lower face exemplifies this imperative. Patient selection and keen analysis must be coupled with an in-depth anatomic understanding for the etiologies of the displeasing features of the heavy neck.

Although the general public seeking facial rejuvenation is increasingly influenced by commercial and corporate interests, treatment protocols must be dictated by diagnosis and safe, reliable outcomes. While procedures labeled as "quick," "mini," "lunch time," and "minimally invasive" have enamored much of the public (thanks in no small part to advertising and marketing campaigns), effective and long lasting treatment for the heavy neck require a commitment on the part of the surgeon and the patient.

The ground work for our modern approach to face lifting in the patient with a heavy neck began in the early 1900s. Bourget, at the Academie de Medicine de Paris presented submental fat removal in 1919, and almost 20 years later described treating platysmal banding.[1] It was Millard, in the late 1960s, who spurned the modern approach to submental lipectomy.[2] Well-known pioneers in facelift procedures, including Tessier,[3] Skoog,[4] Mitz and Peyronie,[3] Lemmon and Hamra,[4] Kamer and colleagues,[5] and McCollough and Pieper,[6] have all helped to delineate the role and various approaches to the superficial musculoaponeurotic system (SMAS) in modern face lifting. It is in the application of various combinations of these techniques, coupled with our detailed anatomic understanding, that today's surgeon is afforded the necessary tools for meaningful rejuvenative treatment of the patient with a heavy neck.

THE IDEAL NECK

The anatomy of the ideal neck defies perfection. In profile, a distinct shadow below the jaw line emanates from a sharp mandibular border, epitomizing the ideal and youthful neck. Perhaps, the most salient feature on lateral view is that of a cervicomental angle approaching ninety degrees.[5] Distinct sternocleidomastoid muscle (SCM) borders should draw the eye from the angle of the mandible to a visible sternal notch. The submental triangle should lie flat and taught. As it extends to the hyoid bone, no convexity should be noted. A slight depression inferior to the hyoid pleasingly accentuates the transition from the cervicomental angle as it approaches the prominence of the thyroid cartilage. Finally, the strong and well-contoured chin sharpens the distinction between the face and neck, resulting in an overall harmonious appearance.

THE HEAVY NECK

Regardless of a person's proximity or lack there of, to one's ideal body weight, the heavy and thick neck stands as a beacon to a discordant appearance. With it, the lean may be mistaken for overweight and the lively for lethargic. Loosened, hanging skin meets the onlooker's eye instantly. It poorly conforms to the contours of the neck

a Department of Otolaryngology, St Vincent's Medical Center, 1 Shircliff Way, Jacksonville, FL 32204, USA
b The Wachholz Clinic, P.A., 2700 Riverside Avenue, Jacksonville, FL 32205, USA
* The Wachholz Clinic, P.A., 2700 Riverside Avenue, Jacksonville, FL 32205.
E-mail address: jhwmd@JAXFACE.com

Facial Plast Surg Clin N Am 17 (2009) 603–611
doi:10.1016/j.fsc.2009.07.002
1064-7406/09/$ – see front matter © 2009 Elsevier Inc. All rights reserved.

structures. This results from reduced elasticity and weakened collagen integrity. Subcutaneous fat in over abundance further obscures the contours of the deeper underlying structures. Significant lipogenesis in the submentum drastically blunts the cervicomental angle. Here, preplatysmal fat is a key culprit. The presence of a low-lying hyoid further accentuates this obtuse angle. Jowling and submandibular fat may serve to blur the distinction between the lower face and neck. With muscular atrophy, the definition of the anterior borders of the SCM and sternal notch are lost. On profile, the cervicomental angle becomes obtuse with laxity of the platysma muscle. Its anterior correlate is seen as vertical neck banding. Overall ptosis of the lower face and neck is further accentuated as the SMAS support thins and weakens. The entirety of the cervical anatomy yields to the downward vector of gravity, exacerbated by the excess weight of the thickened and heavy neck.

Either primary microgenia or an acquired microgenia secondary to bone absorption and dental changes with aging, may greatly increase the discontinuity obvious in the heavy neck. The shape and overall projection of the chin are key components in determining aesthetic treatment strategies. Even a weak chin alone may give the illusion of a short neck as it lessens the distinction from the face to the cervical region.

The culmination of these acquired or congenital factors results in the loss of shadowing beneath the jaw line, and the displeasing bulging of the submental and submandibular triangles. The natural concavity seen in the ideal neck is strikingly absent, having been obliterated by underlying fat. Blunting of the cervicomental angle and any evident vertical muscle banding, further accentuate the unshapely contours. Dedo[7] has described a useful preoperative classification of neck anatomy as it relates to severity in aesthetic appearance based on the level of anatomic involvement of skin, muscle, and bone as it correlates to the overall appearance in neck contour and shape.

SURGICAL TREATMENT OF THE HEAVY FACE AND NECK

As etiology of the heavy neck is multifactorial, its treatment is by nature multimodal. Addressing preplatysmal fat is the cornerstone in rejuvenating the heavy neck. A 2 to 3 cm incision just posterior to the submental crease allows excellent direct visualization and evaluation of the adiposity. Liposuction-cannula dissection (before vacuum connection) is a quick and hemostatic means to undermining the anterior and mid portions of the cervical region.

This maneuver may be followed by performing liposuction with graduated cannula sizes (5–2 mm). The suction cannula aperture must be adjacent to the deeper layer of preplatysmal fat, and not directed toward the under surface of the skin. This is done to help prevent unnatural stippling.

Following submental lipectomy and liposuction (**Fig. 1**), additional fat is removed from the lateral neck. This procedure is done in a supraplatysmal plane with liposuction cannulas, remaining at or below the inferior border of the mandible.

Redundant and excessive adipose tissue in the mentum may be addressed next. Because of the fibrous nature of these retaining mandibular ligaments,[8] we find sharp scalpel and scissor dissection to be superior to cannula liposuction. It is at this point, if chin augmentation is indicated, that a horizontal incision of the mentalis muscle fibers will permit subperiosteal pocket formation. Excellent preformed silicone chin and combination prejowl implants are available and techniques are well described by others (**Fig. 2**).[9,10]

Platysmal cording or banding noted preoperatively should be addressed next. On occasion, the patient who has a heavy neck and exhibits a significantly obtuse cervicomental angle will not have readily discernible platysmal bands on initial examination. However, following submental liposuction, midline platysma nondecussation, laxity, or muscle redundancy may become apparent intraoperatively. Treatment is indeed indicated, as addressing the submental and anterior neck portions of the platysma muscle is paramount (see **Fig. 1**).

Wide undermining in the subcutaneous plane in the anterior neck precedes platysmal maneuvers. Sharp and blunt scissor dissection releases any skin attachments that would hinder smooth redraping. Typically, this extends from mandible to cricoid in the heavy neck. This may be joined with lateral neck undermining during rhytidectomy. Healthy nonsmokers are ideal candidates for these long flaps. Next, the medial edges of the platysma are sharply undermined for approximately 2 cm. Once mobilized along the full extent from mentum to the cricoid or below, subplatysmal fat can be addressed, if necessary.

In the significantly heavy neck, subplatysmal fat may be a contributing factor (see **Fig. 1**). When present, the anterior belly of the digastric muscle should mark its most lateral extent. Resection of this deeper adipose tissue should remain superficial to the mylohyoid muscle. Care must be taken in this area as it may be quite vascular. Judicious removal is key, as over-resection will result in an unnatural (and often uncorrectable) submental depression. While Ramirez advocates plication of the digastric muscle in certain instances (Oscar

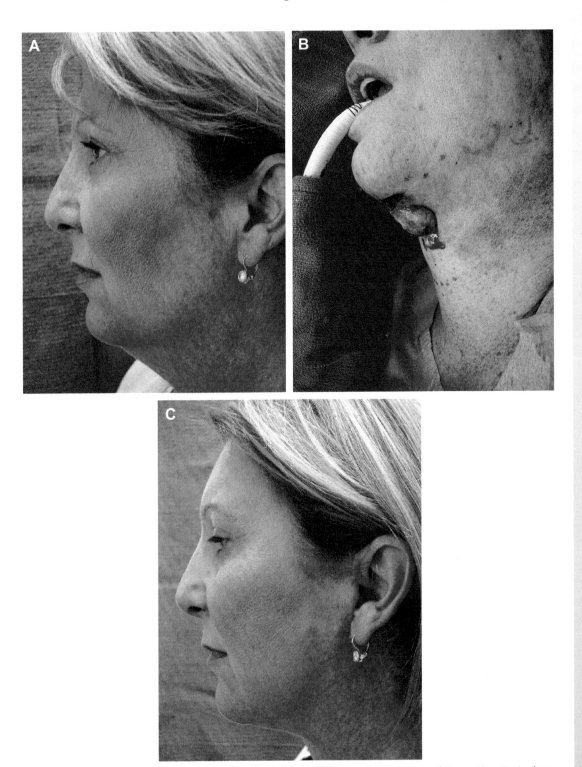

Fig. 1. (*A*) Preoperative view. (*B*) Intraoperative view following submental lipectomy and liposuction. Excised pre- and subplatysmal fat with adjoining vertical edge of platysma muscle, displayed on skin. (*C*) Three month postoperative view following facelift including extensive submental lipectomy and liposuction, combined with platysma plication.

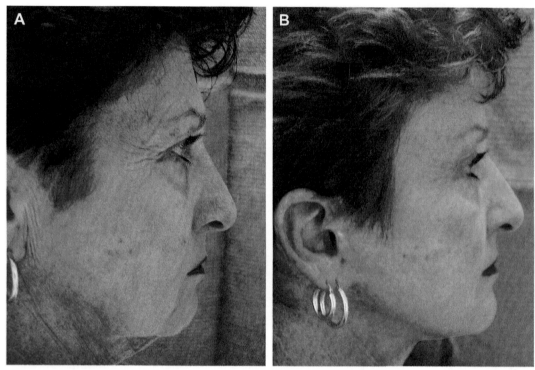

Fig. 2. (*A*) Preoperative view. (*B*) One year postoperative view following facelift, brow lift, chin implant, and platysma plication.

Ramirez, MD, personal communication, 2007), we have not found this to be necessary.

Redundant edges of the platysmal muscle should now be excised conservatively, avoiding any tension on re-approximation. Plication may then proceed from mentum to thyroid cartilage, or more inferiorly, to the cricoid, depending on neck anatomy and desired outcomes. Important surgical pearls include taking muscle edge suture bites of at least 1 cm that include deeper fascia for greater hold and avoidance of pull-through. These knots should be well buried.

Horizontal incisions into the muscle, if indicated, may be performed at this time. When done conservatively, these extend no more than 1 to 2 cm in length, just at or below the inferior extent of plication. Partial or complete transection is thought to (1) alleviate tension along medial closure; (2) allow the platysma to shift superiorly, deepening the cervicomental angle; and (3) reduce the possibility of dual platysmal edges being converted to a noticeable single band following plication (**Figs. 3** and **4**).[8]

Complete transection of the platysma is now less favored than in the past, as bunching deformities and noticeable muscle edge irregularities may result.[5,11,12] However, complete transection may be considered in the patient with an extremely short, fat, and heavy neck in whom the

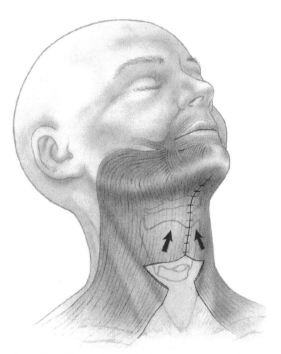

Fig. 3. The effects of partial platysma resection. (*Adapted from* Baker TJ, Gordon HL, Stuzin JM. Rhytidectomy. In: Surgical rejuvenation of the face. St Louis (MO): Mosby; 1996. p. 295.)

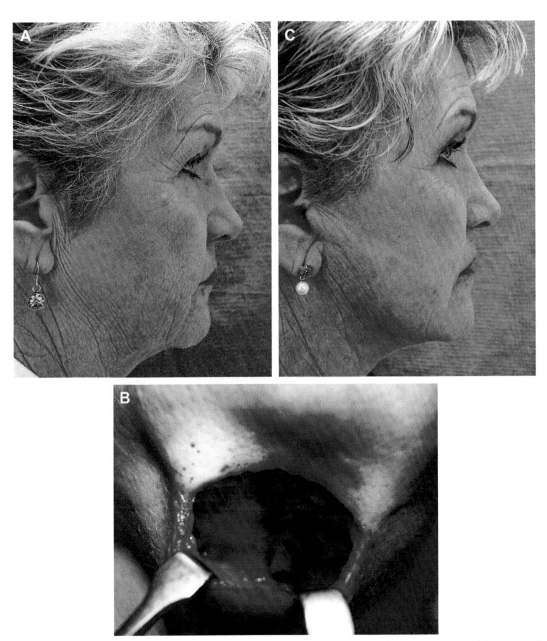

Fig. 4. (*A*) Preoperative view. (*B*) Intraoperative view of submental exposure and platysma treatment. (*C*) Two month postoperative view following facelift with partial anterior platysma transection and plication, and brow lift.

combination of liposuction, platysma plication, partial horizontal myotomy, and rhytidectomy with superior cervical suspension have failed to produce a well-defined contour. The goal of neck contouring is to provide a clear transition from the jaw line to achieving a thinner neck. Some advocate an oblique transection extending from the facial SMAS dissection, paralleling the anterior border of the SCM. If the level of dissection remains well below the jaw line, one avoids placing the marginal mandibular nerve in jeopardy. Once

reaching the anterior neck, the transection is joined with the horizontal myotomy at the level of the cricoid (**Fig. 5**).[8]

An alternative approach that may be applied to the heavy neck is suture suspension. This technique, as described by Giampapa, provides long-term, significant improvement within the neck, especially for the cervicomental angle and mandibular border definition. This is achieved through midline platysmal vertical excision and plication, followed by an interlocking, nonabsorbable suture

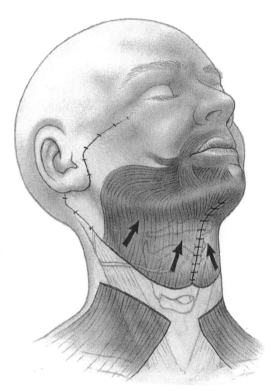

Fig. 5. Following transection of the platysma, the muscle is seen to gap several centimeters. This superior shifting of the platysma will deepen the cervicomental angle and better define the jaw line. (*Adapted from* Baker TJ, Gordon HL, Stuzin JM. Rhytidectomy. In: Surgical rejuvenation of the face. St Louis (MO): Mosby; 1996. p. 297.)

extending from the midline to the mastoid fascia bilaterally.[13] Other similar suspension techniques have used various materials, such as expanded polytetrafluoroethylene (Gortex) to create a sling effect. While indeed these may be long lasting, potentials for infection or visible irregularities must be taken into consideration (Stephen Perkins, MD, personal communication, 2008).

Having addressed the anterior neck directly, one proceeds with the SMAS portion of rhytidectomy. Development of either an extended SMAS flap or deep plane approach may optimize improvement for the patient who has a heavy neck. The platysma of the neck inferior to the mandible is not typically elevated with the exception of its midline contributions. Hamra stresses the importance of avoiding any posterior or lateral tension that may oppose the midline plication. Additionally, he advocates dissecting the superior portions of the platysma while elevating the face lift flap. Care must be exercised in avoiding branches of the facial nerve traversing anteriorly. The facial portion of the platysma above the jaw line is suspended with

a superior vector, otherwise known as posterior platysmaplasty. This maneuver is performed in an attempt to further define the jaw line, and reduce medial banding and bunching (**Fig. 6**).[12]

Others have advocated dividing the inferior portion of the excess SMAS following mobilization. This is done in the infralobular area and can be transposed postauricularly. Again, if using this maneuver, one must be mindful of achieving a more superior vector, to reduce any opposing tension on the midline cervical platysmaplasty (**Fig. 7**).[8]

With rhytidectomy suspension complete, excess skin must then be addressed. Extended skin incisions into the posterior hair line approaching the occiput may be helpful in treating the patient with extreme cervical skin redundancy.[14] While some have advocated creating an incision in a complete circumoccipital manner,[15] we have not found this to be necessary (**Fig. 8**).

No doubt, it is well accepted that neck laxity, adiposity, and vertical banding, as seen in the patient who has a heavy neck, is most aesthetically treated through a submental access combined with the rotation and advancement accomplished in rhytidectomy. With this

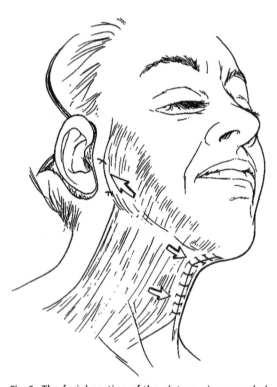

Fig. 6. The facial portion of the platysma is suspended with a more superior vector. Accentuation of the mandibular border is achieved while avoiding a directly opposing force on the midline platysma plication. (*Adapted from* Hamra ST. Composite rhytidectomy. Plast Reconstr Surg 1992;90:1–1.)

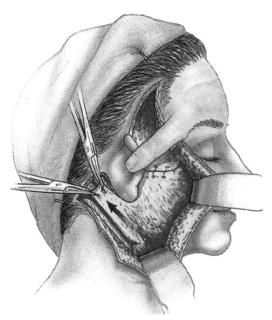

Fig. 7. Following SMAS re-draping in the cheek, the excess SMAS is transposed posterior to the ear to affect contour in the submental and submandibular region by tightening the platysma. The flap is secured to the mastoid fascia. (*Adapted from* Baker TJ, Gordon HL, Stuzin JM. Rhytidectomy. In: Surgical rejuvenation of the face. St Louis (MO): Mosby; 1996. p. 260.)

approach, little if any skin needs to be trimmed at the submental incision, thus avoiding potential bowstringing and contractures.[5] Direct excision submentoplasty, nonetheless, may be considered for the patient whose only isolated concern is submental laxity and fullness and who is reticent to consider rhytidectomy. Some of the more recent contributions to this technique include the T-Z plasty,[16] W-plasty,[17] and vertical ellipse with a T-closure by Farrior.[18] These direct excisional approaches are best suited for aging males, as an external neck scar remains.

Regardless of the technique or approaches chosen, a thorough preoperative discussion with the patient who has a heavy face and neck is vital. Technical challenges and anticipated outcomes should be outlined thoroughly. This is especially crucial in patients requiring large amounts of cervical and submental fat removal. A small subset of this group may even require addressing residual and excess laxity. For these patients, a short-interval, secondary face lift involving skin dissection only, may be appropriate.[19]

SUMMARY: SURGICAL MANAGEMENT OF THE HEAVY FACE AND NECK

The surgical management of the patient who has a heavy lower face and neck requires appreciation

of the multiple anatomic and physiologic factors responsible for the associated displeasing appearance. Preoperative planning and patient selection are key components in achieving optimal outcomes. Furthermore, while approaches and techniques applied in traditional facelifting are beneficial, additional, or modified maneuvers are often necessary to produce the desired outcomes in this challenging patient group.

Areas of special attention include the submentum and anterior neck. While aggressive lipectomy and liposuction are indicated, one must be cautious to avoid skeletonization in this region. This is particularly relevant in treating subplatysmal fat; over-resection results in unnatural and often uncorrectable concavities. In the author's experience, supported by the literature, excision of lax or redundant platysma muscle edges in the midline, followed by meticulous plication and well-placed horizontal myotomies, are the cornerstone in achieving pleasing neck contours.

The question as to which facelift technique (SMAS, extended SMAS, Composite, or deep plane) may be the most efficacious in treating the heavy neck, is yet to be answered. Some contend no perceptible advantages exist with more extensive techniques.[20] Others have presented evidence indicating advantages may exist with a deep-plane approach.[21,22] One technical point is clear: cervical rhytidectomy suspension with a predominantly superior vector will serve to sharpen the jaw line and crisply define the face-to-neck transition. Additionally, by avoiding a posterior, opposing force on the lateral portions of the cervical platysma and SMAS, the midline neck and anterior platysma maneuvers are complemented and reinforced. Lastly, through direct visualization and palpation, the adept surgeon must be certain to preserve an adequate and even thickness of subcutaneous fat on the undersurface of the flap. This helps achieve pleasing re-draping, accentuating the changes affected with the deeper-neck structure techniques, while still preserving the natural shape and architecture of the skin. The outcome affords the patient who has a heavy neck the more desirable contours and features seen in the ideal neck.

As a final note, we are witnessing increasing popularity of bariatric procedures; hence, the number of patients who have undergone bariatric surgery and are seeking facial rejuvenation is on the rise. This group may require special consideration from a medical and surgical standpoint.[23] Management of this subpopulation, with features of excess cervical tissue and adiposity, may require further advancement

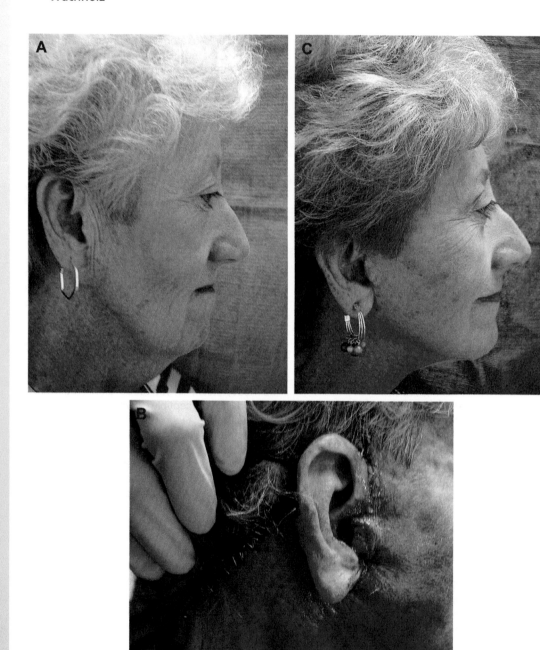

Fig. 8. (A) Preoperative view. (B) Immediate postoperative view illustrating extension of incision into posterior hairline to address significant cervical skin laxity. (C) Two month postoperative view following rhytidectomy with facial platysma suspension, submental lipectomy and liposuction, extended midline plication and partial anterior platysma transection, and brow lift.

of our present surgical techniques. Indubitably, in treating the patient who has a heavy face and neck, one certainty prevails: the surgeon who maintains a diverse armamentarium of skills and techniques will be best equipped to achieve consistently gratifying and reliable outcomes.

REFERENCES

1. Marchac D. Julien Bourguet: the pioneer in aesthetic surgery of the neck. Clin Plast Surg 1983;10:363–5.
2. Millard DR Jr, Pigott RH, Hedo A. Submandibular lipectomy. Plast Reconstr Surg 1968;41:513–22.

3. Mitz V, Peyronie M. The superficial musculoaponeurotic system (SMAS). Plast Reconstr Surg 1976;58:80–8.

4. Lemmon ML, Hamra ST. Skoog rhytidoplasty: a five year experience with 577 patients. Plast Reconstr Surg 1980;65:283–92.

5. Kamer FM, Pieper PG. Surgical treatment of the aging neck. Facial Plast Surg 2001;17(2):123–8.

6. McCollough EG, Perkins SW, Langsdon PR. SAS-MAS suspension rhytidectomy. Rationale and long term experience. Arch Otolaryngol Head Neck Surg 1989;115(2):228–34.

7. Dedo DD. A preoperative classification of the neck for cervicofacial rhytidectomy. Laryngoscope 1980; 90(11):1894–6.

8. Baker TJ, Gordon HL, Stuzin JM. Rhytidectomy. In: Hurley R, editor. Surgical rejuvenation of the face. St. Louis (MO): Mosby; 1996. p. 215–383.

9. Mittleman H. The anatomy of the aging mandible and its importance to facelift surgery. Facial Plast Surg Clin North Am 1994;2:301–11.

10. Glasgold AI, Glasgold MJ. Mentoplasty. Facial Plast Surg Clin North Am 1994;2(3):285–99.

11. Guerrosantos J, Sandoval M, Salazaar J. Long term study of complications of neck lift. Clin Plast Surg 1983;10:563–72.

12. Hamra ST. Neck. In: Hamra ST, editor. Composite rhytidectomy. St. Louis (MO): Quality Medical Publishing; 1993. p. 66–71.

13. Giampapa V, Bitzos I, Ramirez O, et al. Long-term results of suture suspension platysmaplasty for neck rejuvenation: a 13 year follow-up evaluation. Aesthetic Plast Surg 2005;29:332–40.

14. Campbell JP, McCollough EG, Metzinger SE. Posterior cervical rhytidectomy: a valuable adjunct in facial rejuvenation surgery. Otolaryngol Head Neck Surg 1997;116(1):79–90.

15. Marshak H, Morrow DM. "The Stork Lift": a circumoccipital extended neck lift. Aesthetic Plast Surg 2008; 32:850–5.

16. Cronin TD, Biggs TM. The T-Z-plasty for the male "turkey gobbler". Plast Reconstr Surg 1971;47:534–8.

17. Ehlert TK, Thomas JR, Becker FF. Submental W-plasty for correction of "turkey gobbler" deformity. Arch Otolaryngol Head Neck Surg 1990;116:714–7.

18. Bitner JB, Friedman O, Farrior RT, et al. Direct submentoplasty for neck rejuvenation. Arch Facial Plast Surg 2007;9:194–200.

19. Wolfe SA, Fusi S. Treatment of the particular fatty neck and short-interval secondary facelift. Aesthetic Plast Surg 1991;15:195–201.

20. Ivy EJ, Lorenc JP, Aston SJ. Is there a difference? A prospective study comparison lateral and standard SMAS face lifts with extended SMAS and composite rhytidectomies. Plast Reconstr Surg 1996;98:1135–43.

21. Litner JA, Adamson PA. Limited vs. extended facelift techniques: objective analysis of intraoperative techniques. Arch Facial Plast Surg 2006;8:186–90.

22. Kamer FM, Frankel AS. SMAS rhytidectomy versus deep plane rhytidectomy: an objective comparison. Plast Reconstr Surg 1996;102:878–81.

23. Sclafani AP. Restoration of the neck and jaw line after bariatric surgery. In: Fedok F, Nolst Trenite GJ, Becker DG, et al, editors. Facial plastic surgery. New York: Thieme Medical; 2005;21: p. 28–32.

Reflections on Aesthetic Facial Surgery in Men

Ross A. Clevens, MD, FACS[a],*, Stephen Prendiville, MD[b]

KEYWORDS

• Male facial cosmetic surgery • Male facelift • Male necklift

The literature on the approach to the aging face generally centers on the care of the female patient. Most rejuvenating facial aesthetic surgery is performed on women; however, several social and demographic trends have led to an ever-increasing level of interest in facial cosmetic surgery among men. This article focuses on the panoply of unique considerations related to addressing male patients compared to female patients. The authors argue that the care of male patients is characterized by important differences along each step of the surgical process from the initial consultation to the final visit with the patient. Although numerous articles published here and elsewhere catalog the technical considerations related to cosmetic surgery in men, few works address the nonsurgical aspects coupled with managing and connecting with male patients. Men display a different set of motivations, concerns, and aesthetic ideals compared with women. Men also demonstrate a decision-making process and problem-solving approach that contrasts with that observed among women. These unique differences that set men apart from women compel the facial plastic surgeon to manage male patients differently from female patients.

MEN ARE FROM MARS

In 1992, John Gray authored an important psychological and sociologic analysis of men compared with women. This well-known treatise is entitled "Men Are From Mars, Women Are From Venus." The book asserts the notion that men and women are as different from one another as beings from another planet. Gray uses the mythologic metaphor of men being like the Roman god Mars and women like the Goddess Venus as ideal types. Mars is the god of war, the strongest and most fearsome god. Venus is the goddess of love and beauty. Gray offers suggestions for improving husband-wife relationships by understanding the communication style and needs of the opposite gender; these same principles are applicable to any domain in which interactions take place among men and women. Gray's views facilitate our ability to understand and communicate with the sexes. Communication is an integral component of the patient-surgeon relationship. This skill enables us to connect with our patients and guide them through the surgical process to a mutually beneficial conclusion.

An example of Gray's theories is that women complain about problems because they want their problems to be acknowledged, whereas men complain about problems because they are asking for solutions. Women crave listening and understanding, whereas men demand answers. Gray points out that men and women react differently under stress. Men withdraw until they find a solution for their problem. This is referred to as "retreating into their cave." The point of retreating is to take time to determine a solution. Men in their caves are not necessarily focused on the problem at hand. Rather, this is a "time-out" of sorts to allow them to distance themselves from the problems so they can revisit the problem later with a fresh perspective. The process of men's "retreating" to help them to

[a] Clevens Center for Facial Cosmetic Surgery, 1344 South Apollo Boulevard, Suite 100, Melbourne, FL 32901, USA
[b] Southwest Florida Facial Plastic Surgery Associates, 9407 Cypress Lake Drive, Suite A, Fort Myers, FL 33919, USA
* Corresponding author.
E-mail address: info@drclevens.com (R.A. Clevens).

Facial Plast Surg Clin N Am 17 (2009) 613–624
doi:10.1016/j.fsc.2009.06.006
1064-7406/09/$ – see front matter © 2009 Published by Elsevier Inc.

eventually solve a problem contrasts with the natural reaction among women to talk about issues to develop understanding and insight and not necessarily find a solution. This difference leads to the dynamic of men retreating and women seeking to maintain and develop channels of communication. Women nurture while men retreat.

This striking set of differences between what men and women seek in their relationships and styles of communications has direct applicability to male cosmetic surgery patients compared to female patients. "Men Are From Mars, Women Are From Venus" is an important handbook to ease our interactions with our female and male patients and counterparts. The methods of listening and problem solving that we use with our female patients is not necessarily transferable to our male patients. What our male patients are asking us to achieve may be different from what our female patients seek to achieve. Similarly, our listening and problem-solving skills as male surgeons do not naturally transfer to an understanding and empathetic view that enables us to connect with our patients.

The book "Men Are From Mars, Women Are From Venus" presents itself as a means to improving interactions between men and women and getting what you want in your communications and relationships with the opposite sex. This article addresses the variations in positive communication between cosmetic surgeons and male patients versus methods of communication between cosmetic surgeons and female patients.

DEMOGRAPHIC TRENDS IN COSMETIC SURGERY

There has been a dramatic shift in demographic trends related to cosmetic surgery over time. The American Society of Plastic Surgeons (ASPS) poll conducted in 2008 demonstrated a remarkable convergence over time in attitudes among men and women toward cosmetic surgery. The poll revealed that 56% of women and 57% of men approve of cosmetic surgery. More than 30% of women would consider cosmetic surgery for themselves, whereas nearly 20% of men would consider cosmetic surgery for themselves. Interestingly, a nearly equal percentage (almost 80% of men and women) acknowledged that they would not be embarrassed about having cosmetic surgery. It is surprising that the overall level of acceptance and interest in cosmetic surgery is nearly equal between men and women across so many dimensions, yet men comprise a substantially smaller proportion of aesthetic surgery patients.

Attitudes toward facelift surgery in men have shifted dramatically over the last several decades. In the 1970s and 1980s, only 6% to 10% of men admitted to even considering facelift surgery. In the 1990s, this cohort increased to only approximately 12%. The first decade of the twenty-first century (2001–2009) has seen a near doubling in the interest level in facelift surgery among men to more than 20%. Despite these trends in attitudes among men toward cosmetic surgery, men still comprise a stark minority of facial cosmetic surgery patients. There must be an impediment or barrier that bridges the gap between the number of men who state that they are accepting of cosmetic surgery and the actual number of men who seek cosmetic surgery. Perhaps some of these men have retreated to their caves as they contemplate rejuvenating surgery.

These data suggest that the overall level of interest and acceptance of cosmetic surgery among men has nearly tripled over the past decades. We tend to underestimate the cohort of male patients among our potential patient pool. Men merit greater attention and focus in our facial plastic surgery practices so that we can connect with this population.

CONSULTATION WITH MALE COSMETIC SURGERY PATIENTS

Experience demonstrates that men often present to our offices for consultation in a somewhat different manner than women. Whereas women generally schedule their own consultation themselves, men often ask their spouse or significant other to schedule the consultation on their behalf. This approach represents apprehension or discomfort on the part of men in expressing their aesthetic concerns and misgivings. Men are more likely to follow their spouse's lead into cosmetic surgery. Men often elect aesthetic surgery after their spouse has already done so, which further suggests some degree of reluctance or lack of comfort in initiating cosmetic surgery care. Although poll data suggest that men are nearly as comfortable as women in seeking cosmetic surgery, in reality there seems to be a greater degree of hesitancy in taking the first steps toward surgery. In our experience, a supportive husband sitting by his wife at the consultation adds himself on to his spouse's scheduled consult. This is known as the "Oh, by the way Doc…" scenario in which the man piggybacks on his wife's appointment. Alternatively, a woman turns to her male companion and asks, "What about…" drawing forth his aesthetic concerns in a disarming fashion.

Men show a strong tendency toward Internet and email consultation and communication throughout their care. We have received preconsultation emails with simple direct statements as, "I know that it's time. I am ready for a facelift." Men are much more apt to send postoperative emails concerning wound care, whereas women are generally more likely to come to the office for evaluation of specific concern. The initial inquiry with the practice is more likely to come through a nondirect resource such as the Internet, as compared with telephone or face-to-face inquires. Male patients tend to reschedule more often than female counterparts before actually coming in for the initial consultation. Men tend to have a much higher no-show rate throughout their course of care, from initial consultation through postoperative care. This should not necessarily be viewed as a negative indicator; rather it seems to be an intrinsic characteristic of male patients.

When a man schedules an appointment for his consultation, usually he has made up his mind in advance and is ready to schedule surgery. To borrow Gray's verbiage, once the man emerges from his cave, he is ready for action. Male patients are often more reluctant to discuss their motivations and reasons for seeking cosmetic surgery. Whereas female patients may be compelled or comforted to share their thoughts and feelings about why they are compelled to seek cosmetic surgery, men are unmotivated to express their views. Men more commonly state their concerns outright without reference to contributing emotional or social components. Men tend to be more direct and to the point with regard to their desired outcome. Consultations with men tend to be much more focused and shorter in duration as compared with the typical initial consultation with women. These observations on the initial inquiry in men provide not only guidance on how to handle the male patient but also methods to connect with prospective males patient seeking cosmetic surgery. Just as men may have "emerged from their cave" with the decision to move forward with cosmetic surgery without much further discussion, women may need to discuss the options and dynamics of cosmetic surgery at much greater length before making a decision.

During the consultation, men are less likely to share their impetus for seeking rejuvenating surgery. Some express concerns related to the workplace or personal relationships. As is typical with men, they seem to be less willing to share their life experience as it relates to their desire for cosmetic surgery compared with women. An alternative explanation is that men are less connected with their motivation for turning to aesthetic surgery. Men seem less anxious than women, yet this appearance is merely a contrast between the sexes in their ability to appreciate their own anxieties. This may represent a return to the cave for the man as compared with the capacity for the wave of compassion that women possess.

FACTORS IN MALE DECISION MAKING

During the consultation, we aim to keep it simple and straight with men, getting to the point more directly and with less pomp. Men often present with a list of bullet points that concern them. The typical consultation with men is shorter in duration than with women. Although men are often apparently directed and decisive about their direction, it seems that in the end men rely more on their surgeon's judgment than women. Men tend to take more of an executive approach to decision making, relying on their choice of surgeon and then delegating to that surgeon the decision-making authority. Men are less swayed by the impressions of friends in regard to cosmetic surgery than women.

The consultation with male candidates tends to be focused and purpose driven. Many men express a narrower scope of concern than women. Some men are more easily satisfied with the results of one directed procedure than multiple procedures. Typical female aging face patients consider the gestalt of the outcome with respect to their overall appearance, whereas men tend to be more focused. Female patients grasp the impact of a complete aesthetic makeover, whereas men are more directed and purpose driven. In other words, women are often most pleased if we address as many of their aging concerns in one setting where possible and "hit a home run." Women are more likely to see the disharmony or imbalance in partial sets of procedures than men. Women may seek a facelift to rejuvenate the midface, jaw line, and neck, whereas men are more likely to be concerned with a narrower area of focus, such as the submental region. It is more common to perform more limited procedures in men and "hit a single or double." For example, a man concerned with his neckline may opt for a direct necklift or limited necklift, whereas a woman would instead seek a complete facelift. The ability of limited-incision or direct necklift procedures to adequately address the concerns of patients and alternative treatments should be discussed carefully. Men tend to focus on a specific concern: "I don't like my turkey wattle, but I don't care about my jowls," or "I don't like my baggy upper and lower eyelids, but I don't care about my crow's feet." These dichotomous sentiments are rarely heard among women (**Figs. 1–6**).

Often men have a more limited window of time that they are willing to dedicate to aesthetic surgery than women. Men tend to weigh outcome versus downtime far more than women. Men may dedicate 1 week of recovery time to a limited neck-lift but not 2 to 3 weeks of downtime to a facelift. This calculus that applies such weight to downtime to the potential relative detriment of overall outcome is less commonly observed among our female patients. As noted, men tend to be more focused in their concerns and tend to accept more limited procedures that directly address their concerns. They are less easily persuaded to add supplementary procedures that may improve their outcome. This obstacle requires more educational effort than in women. Men exhibit a greater degree of indecisiveness early in their decision making and tend to focus more on monetary concerns, but once settled on a decision, men tend to be more directed. With respect to financial concerns, men need more positive reinforcement in a more incisive way than women. Men tend to demonstrate buyer's remorse, which may lead to a change of heart in terms with moving forward with the procedure. Although men demonstrate this degree of indecisiveness, they are less likely to come in for a second consultation than women and are

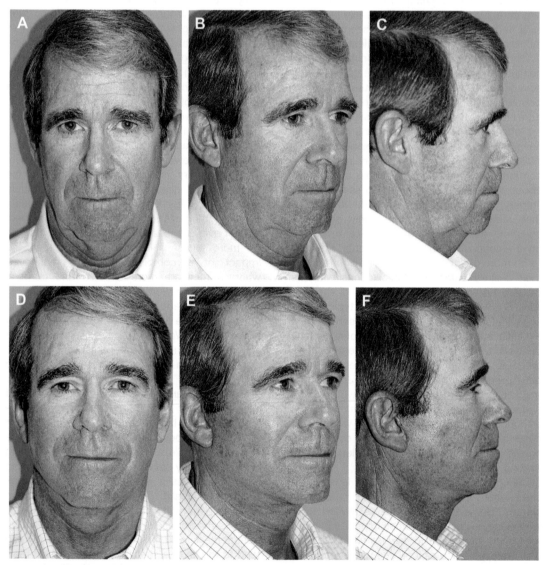

Fig. 1. This 52-year-old engineer sought complete facial rejuvenation after expressing concerns with aging changes related to the lower two thirds of the face and neck. Facelift was performed to address these findings.

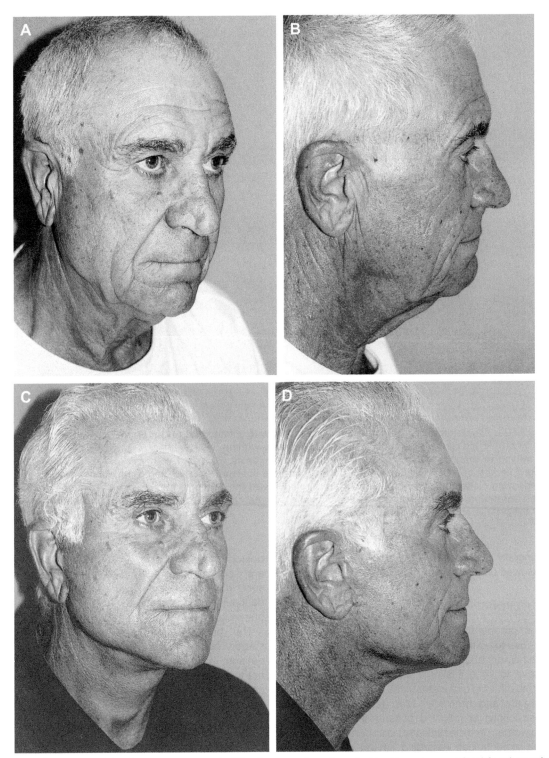

Fig. 2. This 69-year-old retiree was concerned with a heavy neck and weak chin. He underwent facelift enhanced with a chin-jowl implant. As is so often the case in male facelift surgery, this patient's wife is also a longstanding patient of the practice and previous facelift patient.

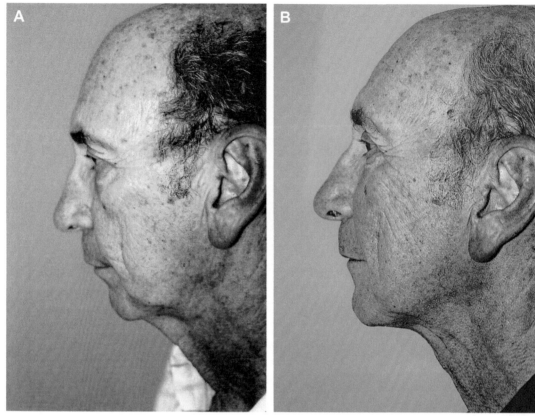

Fig. 3. This 73-year-old real estate professional presented with a limited set of concerns. Specifically, he objected to his profile and marked neck laxity. He was not concerned with his cheek, midface, or jowls. This gentleman was unwilling to consider the prolonged recovery time commitment associated with cervicofacial rhytidectomy. A direct necklift or submentoplasty was performed with the direct anterior excision of redundant neck skin with underlying platysmaplasty. This focused procedure addressed the patient's limited scope of concerns within his time constraints as related to recovery commitment. Of note, this patient's wife is also a longstanding patient of the practice and previous facelift patient.

generally more pleased to have their concerns resolved on the phone.

PERIOPERATIVE PATIENT EDUCATION

The preoperative teaching visit with men also tends to differ from the visit with women. Remember that men seek solutions. With men, strive to keep it simple and drive to the point. Stress the logic of instructions. Answer questions directly and precisely. Men tend not to read instructions or follow directions as meticulously as women. In male patients it is important to stress the expectations regarding limited activity after surgery. We more clearly stress the postoperative activity level and anticipated recovery course so that men feel comfortable with the expectations for limited activity after surgery. In our practice, we have found that men are more comfortable with care given by a single nurse during their

postoperative visits. In our practice we assign a specific nurse to each male patient so that he sees the same nurse each time to reinforce continuity and minimize obstacles to clear communication.

The postoperative care of male aesthetic surgery patients differs from the care of female patients in numerous important ways. Men tend not to follow instructions as carefully or as clearly as women. It is important to get to the point and stress the key considerations in aftercare. Men tend not to tolerate discomfort well, yet they deny the need for postoperative pain medications. This is associated with anxiety and elevation in blood pressure, which may predispose to postoperative bleeding, hematoma formation, and bruising. Men are often too quick to return to work and higher activity levels; it is important to monitor their activity during the postoperative period. In our experience, men tend to be less

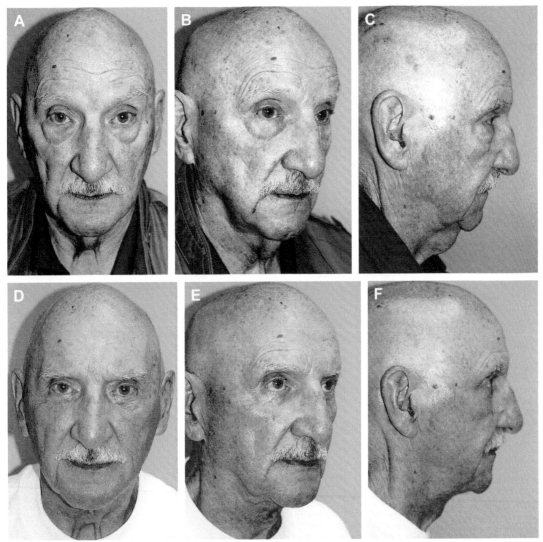

Fig. 4. This 78-year-old entertainer sought rejuvenation of the neck. A direct necklift or submentoplasty was performed with the direct anterior excision of neck skin with underlying platysmaplasty. This procedure exceeded the patient's expectations relative to outcome within a limited postoperative time frame.

diligent with the aftercare of wounds, so closer follow-up in the office is indicated to facilitate favorable healing. A bowel regimen may be necessary to prescribe after surgery, especially in male patients. It is important to avoid straining and Valsalva after surgery because they can be associated with bleeding. Men tend to avoid some of their follow-up appointments and tend not to follow up properly, or at least according to our schedule. Men, however, are quick to call the office with questions, which should be addressed as fully as possible at the time of their inquiry, recognizing that the men are less likely to follow-up at their next scheduled visit. Men tend to feel secure with the continuity of one nurse who can act as their concierge and remain their contact source throughout their facelift experience.

PERIOPERATIVE COSMETIC SURGERY CONSIDERATIONS

Male facelift surgery differs from aging face surgery in women in several important ways, such as careful incision placement that preserves the hair pattern, techniques to manage the heavy neck, and unique considerations in avoiding postoperative complications.

Preserving the hair pattern is important in male and female patients. Hairline incisions beveled parallel to the hair follicles avoid incisional

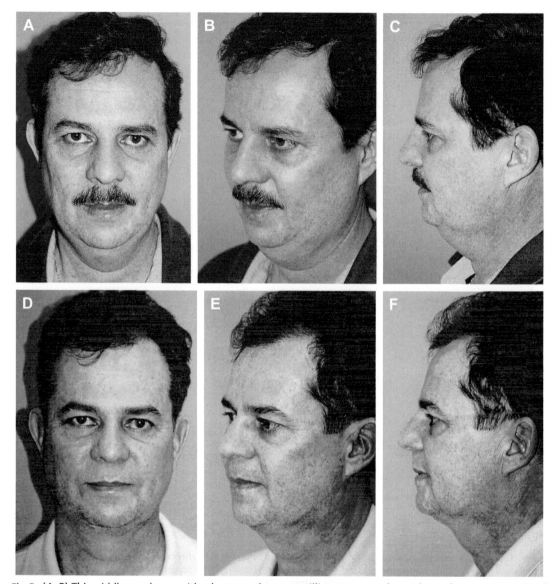

Fig. 5. (*A–D*) This middle-aged man with a heavy neck was unwilling to accept the prolonged recovery associated with facelift and did not want an anterior neck scar. Instead, he elected for a limited necklift approach comprised of cervicofacial liposuction and underlying platysmaplasty without the direct excision of skin. This procedure offers the tradeoff of a quick recovery with less scarring but produces a less dramatic result.

alopecia. Avoiding electrocautery of hair follicles further preserves hair-bearing skin. Incisions are best hidden within hair-bearing regions. It is important to recognize that men do not typically wear makeup to camouflage incisions and are not as comfortable altering their hair pattern to hide incisions as are female patients. This makes incision placement and the creation of inconspicuous incisions even more critical in male patients.

Incision design in male patients affords surgeons many challenges. There is no ideal incision, and the placement of the incision is modified in each case depending on the hairline pattern and

an assessment of where the final scars lie after the tissues are mobilized and redraped (**Fig. 7**). The postauricular limb of the facelift incision is best placed on the posterior surface of the ear because of its tendency to migrate posteriorly and inferiorly. This keeps the incision out of view. As the incision passes from the postauricular limb into the occipital region, it should cross the narrowest non–hair-bearing region along the postauricular mastoid skin posterior to the ear. It should be recognized that the pattern of hair-bearing skin within the male beard is altered by facelift surgery. Men should be advised that they may need to shave

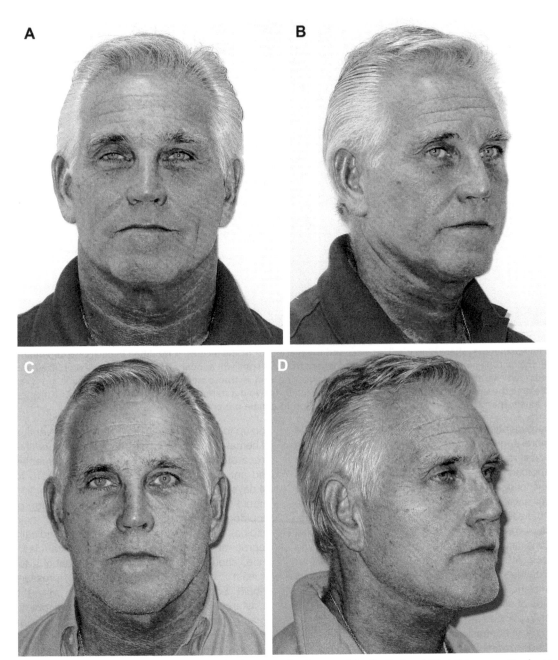

Fig. 6. (*A–D*) A second example of a man with a heavy neck who opted for limited necklift. (*A*) Preoperative front view. (*B*) Preoperative oblique view. (*C*) Postoperative front view. (*D*) Postoperative oblique view.

posterior to the ear after facelift because the skin is transposed into this region. Whereas the facelift incision may be placed in a pretragal or retrotragal location in women, depending on the surgeon's preference, a retrotragal incision in a man would bring the hair-bearing beard skin into the ear canal. Thus, the pretragal placement of the incision is much more common in men. Retrotragal incisions should be reserved for men with darker hair for whom hair-removal techniques, such as intense

pulse light or laser hair removal, are effective. If a retrotragal incision is used, these hair removal techniques and the timeline expected in using them should be discussed preoperatively. In some cases, a hairline margin incision is preferable in men to avoid a stair-stepped occipital hairline or preserve the sideburn.

Because men have thicker skin and heavier muscles than women, the male neck is generally categorized as a "heavy neck." Technical

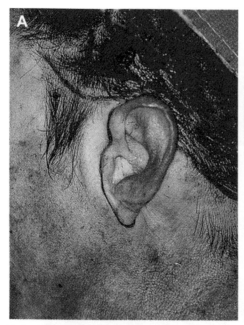 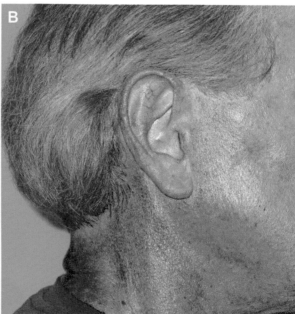

Fig. 7. (*A*) An example of incision placement in a male facelift candidate. Incision design in the male patient offers many challenges. There is no ideal incision, and the placement of the incision is modified in each case depending on the hairline pattern and an assessment of where the final scars will appear after the tissues are mobilized and redraped. Recall that in the male patient, hair-bearing skin is transposed behind the ear. In some cases, to preserve the sideburn, a hairline incision may be elected. To avoid a stepped hairline, an occipital hairline incision is an alternative. (*B*) Example of a retrotragal incision in a male patient.

considerations in addressing the heavy neck include more aggressive surgical defatting and a strong corset anterior platysmaplasty. The deep plane approach may further facilitate mobilization anchoring of the aging tissues. Men exhibit stronger chins with greater anterior projection than women. Whereas geniomandibular hypoplasia is always assessed in the evaluation of the aging face, additional consideration is merited in surgery of the male aging face. Attention focuses on the possible use of an extended anatomic chin implant or a chin-jowl implant. In women, the tendency is to err on the side of either not placing an implant or undersizing an implant so as not to create a masculine appearance. In contrast, the approach to the male patient tends toward considering a chin implant to create a stronger and more angular youthful and masculine contour.

AVOIDING COMPLICATIONS IN MALE FACELIFT SURGERY

Hematoma is the cardinal complication that is observed at a much higher rate in men than in women. Men join smokers and hypertensive patients with a two- to fourfold increased relative risk in hematoma formation compared with female patients. The incidence of expanding or major hematomas is 1.5% to 4% in all facelift patients

and up to 10% to 15% in male patients. Prevention of hematoma is aided by appropriate preoperative preparation of patients. Homeopathic remedies and anticoagulants should be avoided for 10 to 14 days before and after surgery. Special attention should be given to patients on a combination of clopidogrel (Plavix) and acetyl salicylic acid (aspirin). These patients, if deemed medically appropriate for surgery and given medical clearance, should discontinue these medications for at least 2 weeks before surgery. Blood pressure should be controlled perioperatively with the assistance of the patient's primary care practitioner. Use of preoperative oral clonidine, as described in the article on anesthesia in this issue can be a valuable tool in managing blood pressure. There is no substitute for meticulous intraoperative hemostasis, which may be facilitated by normotensive anesthesia to observe for bleeding. The intentional transient elevation of blood pressure before wound closure aids in observing bleeding before conclusion of the operation. Limited subcutaneous dissection in combination with the deep facelift technique diminishes dead space and may be associated with a lower incidence of hematoma formation after facelift surgery. Keen postoperative control of blood pressure, nausea, and vomiting helps to prevent unwanted hypertensive episodes during the perioperative period.

One of the authors (RC) makes generous use of tissue adhesives to facilitate hemostasis and flap adhesion and minimize bruising. Tissue adhesives that facilitate flap adhesion and may aid in hemostasis include platelet-rich plasma (eg, Tisseel, Surgifoam, FloSeal, and Plasmax). Platelet gel, also known as platelet-rich plasma or platelet-enhanced leukocyte-rich gel, is a substance that is created by pheresing platelet-rich plasma from whole blood and combining it with thrombin and calcium or other activators to form a coagulum. This gel may facilitate hemostasis and flap adhesion. Tisseel is a two-component fibrin biomatrix that offers highly concentrated human fibrinogen to seal tissue and stop diffuse bleeding. Surgifoam is an absorbable gelatin sponge comprised of malleable, porcine gelatin intended for hemostatic use by applying to a bleeding surface. FloSeal consists of a bovine-derived gelatin matrix component and thrombin that also functions as a hemostatic agent. The Plasmax system enables the creation of platelet-rich plasma and an autologous fibrin glue and sealant.

Suction drains and pressure dressings are also important in the postoperative management of male facelift patients. In male patients, the compression dressing is removed on the first postoperative and the skin flaps/incisions evaluated. A slightly less compressive dressing is then applied for a second day. Postoperative control of blood pressure, pain, nausea, and vomiting minimizes the likelihood of hematoma formation. Clonidine (0.1–0.2 mg) may be administered on a daily basis for several days after surgery to minimize unwanted elevations in blood pressure and perhaps reduce the incidence of postoperative hematoma formation. Finally, some homeopathic remedies, such as arnica montana and bromelain, may facilitate hemostasis and minimize postoperative bruising.

As discussed elsewhere in this issue, hematoma often presents as increasing pain, pressure, restlessness, and apprehension. The treatment and early recognition of this are important through close postoperative surveillance. Once a hematoma is identified, the patient should be returned promptly to the operating room for evacuation of the hematoma under aseptic conditions. Minor collections may lend themselves to needle aspiration in the office. An untreated and unrecognized hematoma is further complicated by infection, skin necrosis, and unfavorable healing.

LONG-TERM FOLLOW-UP OF MALE COSMETIC SURGERY PATIENTS

In long-term follow-up, men—like women—need positive reinforcement, which is best accomplished in a simple and direct manner. Whereas women are accustomed to skin care, massage, and aesthetic follow-up, men are not. Men are less apt to follow a postoperative skin care regimen to maintain, improve, or enhance their aesthetic outcome. Satisfied male patients tend not to keep their long-term follow-up appointments. If a patient is satisfied, you may never see him again once he has healed. We obtain postoperative photographs earlier and more often in male patients than female patients, recognizing their likelihood not to return for long-term postoperative visits.

DISSATISFIED MALE COSMETIC SURGERY PATIENTS

We all have dissatisfied patients in our practices. To assist in our management of male patients who are dissatisfied, we return to Gray's thoughts on the differences in communication styles between men and women. Remember that women complain about their problems to have their problems appreciated and acknowledged. Women are not necessarily seeking solutions or answers. Instead, women want their concerns heard, recognized, and validated. On the other hand, men complain about problems because they are asking for solutions. Although we tend to see dissatisfied female patients often and listen patiently, surgeons are advised to seek solutions and offer remedies to male patients as early as indicated. This approach addresses directly men's source of concern. All patients, male and female, undergo aesthetic surgery to improve self-image and appearance.

Dissatisfaction may result from surgical complications, unrealistic expectations on the part of the patient, or failure of the surgeon to inform the patient. In all cases it is important to maintain confidence and project a positive outlook. Listen to dissatisfied patients—male and female—and accept their problems. Women benefit from frequent supportive and compassionate visits, whereas men benefit more from solutions that direct their concerns. In either case, respond affirmatively and not defensively. Recognize and share with patients that time improves many concerns.

Given their desire to seek solutions to real or perceived problems, men may follow an entirely different course when dissatisfied with a surgeon. Men are more likely to physically threaten or harm a surgeon when unhappy. Although rare, documented cases exist of men performing violent acts and even killing plastic surgeons who treated them. An interesting anecdote occurred with one of the authors with a male patient (scheduled for a facelift) who was lying on the operating room table, just before the induction of anesthesia. The patient, who previously was a professional gambler in Las Vegas, nonchalantly looked up and stated, "Doctor, I hope that you do a great job, because I don't believe in lawyers...but I do believe in getting even." Needless to say, his concerns were carefully listened to and his needs addressed, and he became a satisfied patient.

Taking a patient from prospective patient to satisfied patient is a three-step process: (1) preoperative consultation, (2) surgical technique, and (3) management of postoperative concerns. In the preoperative consultation, the concerns and motivations of men must be carefully coaxed out and listened to. Because men do not experience and do not often tolerate substantial appearance changes as do women, expected surgical results and image changes must be bluntly described them. Analysis of psychological stability and vigilance for prototypical "red flags," such as the recently divorced ("ready to look good get back on the dating scene") man, are essential. Surgical technique must be modified carefully to accommodate male hair growth characteristics, and a specific effort should be made to avoid feminization of the male jawline with appropriate use of facelift vectors. Because an acute cervicomental angle is a symbol of athletic, masculine appearance, an aggressive approach to the neck is almost mandatory. Postoperative management of male patients is somewhat more complex because of concerns regarding patient follow-up, adherence to postoperative instructions, and ability to express concerns. These characteristics of male patients make it incumbent on the surgeon and staff to be more aggressive in follow-up, via telephone and during office visits, of correct and incorrect behaviors, wound care, and management of expectations. Following this three-step rule is a basic tenant for any form of surgical patient care and is especially important in treatment of men.

SUMMARY

Whereas many article focus on the technical aspects of aesthetic surgery in men, this article addresses some of the nonsurgical considerations in caring for male patients. Although most cosmetic surgery is performed on women, we are witnessing an ever-increasing level of interest in aesthetic surgery among men. With this rise in interest among men, the unique considerations related to addressing male patients compared to female patients merit our attention. The care of male patients is characterized by important differences along each step of the surgical process, from the initial consultation to the final patient visit. Men display a different set of motivations, concerns, and aesthetic ideals compared with women. Men also demonstrate decision-making processes and problem-solving approaches that contrast with approaches observed among women. These unique differences that set men apart from women compel facial plastic surgeons to manage male patients differently from female patients.

Pearls in Facelift Management

Marc S. Zimbler, MD[a],*, Grigoriy Mashkevich, MD[b]

KEYWORDS
- Facelift • Facelift pearls • Rapid recovery facelift
- Preoperative • Management

PREOPERATIVE PEARLS

The preoperative management of a facelift patient sets the stage for a streamlined surgery coupled with a speedy postoperative recovery. Various recommendations are started well before the surgical procedure begins to ensure the best possible results and experience for the patient. Although the surgical result is clearly the most important gauge by which rhytidectomy surgery is measured, one must not underestimate the patient's perspective regarding the surgical experience. This perspective includes anxiety about surgery, postoperative discomfort, and ease of recovery with return to normal daily activities. In many cases, these concerns are some of the most important considerations that prevent patients from undergoing cosmetic surgery. If a patient recovers quickly with minimal bruising, this experience will lead to a high level of satisfaction and in many cases can evolve into the best marketing technique for a surgeon's practice. A surgeon's patients form the strongest practice-building tools, and quick and uneventful recovery from surgery will undoubtedly facilitate patients in encouraging others to come under a particular surgeon's care.

The authors take several steps to ensure a smooth recovery period with outstanding results. Such steps are important in the wound-healing process and also are critical in enabling patients to feel that they are contributing to their own recovery.

The Facelift Consultation

The initial cosmetic consultation with the patient sets the stage for everything that comes thereafter.

Although many physicians believe the consultation begins when they first walk into the room to examine the patient, this is hardly the case. The consultation actually begins well before the physician ever set eyes on the patient and includes the physician's reputation as a surgeon, the physician's relationship with colleagues (other physicians or nurses), bedside manner, Web site, and even the press he or she has received. All these items are measures by which the physician will be evaluated before the patient ever sets foot in the office.

The next critical measure before the actual office consultation is the patient's first interaction with the office, which occurs over the telephone. When the patient calls to schedule, is making the appointment a pleasurable experience? Is it difficult to get through on the phone? Is the patient placed on hold for an extended period of time? If the patient must leave a message, is the call returned promptly? Most importantly, is the staff informative and courteous? Are they able to answer detailed questions about the practice, the physician's medical background and board certification, frequency of performing surgery, and hospital affiliations? All these points, which may seem inconsequential to the average physician, are paramount in the patient's mind when choosing a plastic surgeon.

The next and most critical test is the actual office visit. Again, it is the staff that makes the first impression. When the patient arrives, is the staff friendly an engaging? Is the office well appointed and tastefully decorated (**Fig. 1**)? Is the environment warm and receptive to the patient or cold and sterile like a hospital clinic?

[a] Facial Plastic & Reconstructive Surgery, Department of Otolaryngology-Head & Neck Surgery, Beth Israel Medical Center, 10 Union Square East, Suite 4J, New York, NY 10003, USA
[b] Facial Plastic & Reconstructive Surgery, Department of Otolaryngology-Head & Neck Surgery, The New York Eye & Ear Infirmary, 310 East 14 Street, 6th floor, New York, NY 10003, USA
* Corresponding author.
E-mail address: mzimbler@chpnet.org (M.S. Zimbler).

Facial Plast Surg Clin N Am 17 (2009) 625–632
doi:10.1016/j.fsc.2009.06.011

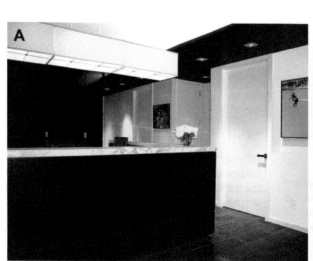
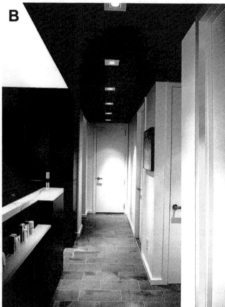

Fig. 1. (*A*) Reception desk and (*B*) hallway in surgeon's office.

In the authors' practices, after the consultation is completed and the patient has decided to move forward with scheduling surgery, the surgical coordinator takes over. The patient is given a medical clearance form to be completed by the primary care physician and detailed preoperative instructions, which the patient takes home to review. Finally, a preoperative visit is set up that occurs 2 weeks before surgery.

Approximately 6 weeks before surgery, the authors like to have many patients start a formal skin care routine, which complements any facial skin tightening surgery. The authors prefer the Obagi Condition & Enhance system (Obagi Medical Products, Long Beach, California) (**Fig. 2**) for surgical procedures with a 0.05% tretinoin regimen. This system is convenient for patients because it is an all-inclusive regimen that is professionally packaged, has a respected brand name, and provides predictable results. The system comes in two forms; the authors prefer the system designated for surgical procedures, which is a milder version of the prior Nu-derm regimen. The authors provide the patient, free of charge, an Obagi travel-pack size. This courtesy helps prepare the skin for surgery and gives patients great results with glowing skin; it also introduces patients to a product that they can continue to use for years after the procedure is completed. Having this constant return of patient flow after surgery will encourage patients to stay in touch with the office and keep abreast of all of the latest technological advances and trends.

Two Weeks Before Surgery

The 2-week window before surgery is a critical period in preparing the patient for a rapid and smooth surgical recovery. This process begins during the ever-important presurgical visit. During this extensive office visit the patient is educated about the mechanics of surgery and the recovery period. During this consultation, all remaining patient questions are answered, and patients are prepared for the upcoming surgical procedure.

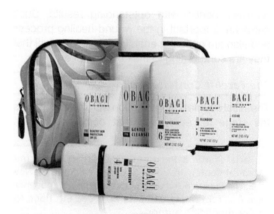

Fig. 2. Obagi skin care products (Obagi Medical Products, Long Beach, California).

Discussion about the surgical process and recovery is a critical step in alleviating much of patients' anxiety. A forthright session serves to set reasonable expectations for patients while putting their minds at ease. Postoperative complications are discussed at length. The authors find it helpful to have patients sign a preprinted complication sheet to ensure that no questions are left unanswered. Many of these preprinted surgery-specific forms can be obtained from colleagues or purchased from medical societies and then customized to one's own practice.

Next, the authors recommend discontinuing the use of any products (whether prescription, over-the-counter, or homeopathic) that may interfere with blood clotting (**Box 1**), as long as their discontinuance is approved by the primary physician. Particular attention must be paid to patients who have chronic conditions such as arthritis, migraine headaches, and low back pain and those who are on long-term medical regimens. For most patients this list includes baby aspirin, various nonsteroidal anti-inflammatory drugs, and/or narcotic combination drugs. Also, many herbal and homeopathic remedies such as green tea or St. John's wort have blood-thinning properties. The use of vitamin E also is discontinued, along with omega-3 fatty acids and fish oils.

Two Days Before Surgery

The authors recommend that patients have all of their prescriptions filled at least 2 days before surgery to prevent any last-minute rush. Typical patient prescriptions include an antibiotic, a painkiller, and some form of anxiolytic (which doubles as a sleeping aid). Patients are given a prescription for Valium in case they become particularly anxious the day before surgery. This prescription also can be used during the postoperative period and in many cases decreases the amount of postoperative narcotic requirements.

All patients are started on a combination of *Arnica Montana*[1] (SINECCH, Alpine Pharmaceuticals) and bromelain[2,3] (500 mg, three times per day) 2 days before surgery to diminish postoperative bruising and swelling. Some physicians also prescribe vitamin K (mephyton, 5 mg), but the authors have not found this to be beneficial.

For patients who color their hair, the authors suggest this be done before surgery because hair chemicals are not permitted for at least 1 month after facelift surgery. It is also recommended that all alcohol use be discontinued at this point before surgery.

Box 1
Commonly prescribed medications and homeopathic remedies known to prolong bleeding time

Patients are asked to stop using these substances 3 weeks before surgery (with appropriate clearance for prescribed medications).

Blood thinners and anti-inflammatory agents

Coumadin

Plavix

Aspirin

Aspirin-containing products

Salicylates

Nonsteroidal anti-inflammatory drugs (Motrin, Advil, Aleve, Ibuprofen, Celebrex, Vioxx, and others)

Over-the-counter pain medications (except Tylenol)

Arthritis medications

Vitamins and dietary supplements

Multivitamins

Vitamin E

Fish oils

Omega-3 fatty acids

St. John's wort

Ginkgo biloba

Garlic

Ginger

Papaya

Chamomile

Ginseng

Green tea

The Day Before Surgery

Several things happen the day before surgery to alleviate any presurgical jitters the patient might have and to instill comfort and confidence in the surgical team. First, the authors' staff always calls the patient to review their preoperative instructions and answer any last-minute questions. During this conversation the oral intake status, preoperative medications, and postoperative private-duty nursing arrangements are reviewed. It is amazing how many little details are caught during this simple telephone conversation that potentially could cause a delay in surgery. Finally, the authors always speak personally with the patient the evening before surgery to let the patient know how enthused they are about the procedure and to reassure them that every precaution will be taken to ensure their safety and comfort. These telephone calls require minimal effort from the physician and staff; however, they go a long way in solidifying patient confidence and comfort.

INTRAOPERATIVE PEARLS
Holding-Area Basics

The authors make sure they arrive well before surgery to allow adequate time with the patient, nursing, and anesthesia. On the morning of surgery, they also spend a few solitary moments in a unhurried manner reviewing the patient's chart and focusing on the medical history, requested surgical procedure, photographs, and personal preferences. It is very important not to appear rushed, short tempered, or disorganized before surgery.

The surgeon should personally and legibly complete the consent form to avoid any confusion in the operating room. Some physicians prefer to use preprinted consent forms specific for each surgical procedure, thereby documenting all pertinent issues in advance of surgery. Many of these forms can be quite lengthy and detailed. The authors believe it is best to review them in the physician's office before surgery, rather than in the holding area where patients may feel rushed and unable to ask all their questions.

The authors ensure the availability of all supplies required for marking the patient before surgery. These items include the correct marking pen, calipers, rulers, hair clips, and other devices. Some surgical facilities may not have the exact supplies; therefore, inquiring in advance may prevent

unnecessary aggravation and delays. The authors prefer to perform partial markings while the patient is sitting upright in the holding area (actual preauricular markings are made in the operating room). They find it particularly helpful to mark out several specific areas, including the malar high point, jowls, nasolabial folds, cervicomental angle, platysmal bands, mandibular angle, and submental crease (**Fig. 3**). In many instances, when the patient is supine on the surgical table, these landmarks can become obscured. Some surgeons also like to prepare the hair in the holding area, but the authors find this step to be time consuming and uncomfortable for the patient. It is much simpler and quicker to prepare the hair after the patient is sedated on the operating table.

Induction and Patient Positioning

Effective communication with the anesthesiologist begins with a discussion regarding the level of anesthesia required for the procedure. The type and depth of anesthesia depends on numerous factors, including preferences of the surgeon and anesthesiologist, operative setting, length of procedure, and patient's comfort level. If general endotracheal anesthesia is selected, the type and placement of the endotracheal tube should be clarified with the anesthesiologist. This communication contributes significantly to optimal and safe airway management for the duration of the procedure. The authors prefer an oral RAE endotracheal tube, placed and fixed in the midline to the upper incisors with surgical sutures. The tube is not taped, because taping would restrict the tube's mobility and the surgeon's access to submental region, particularly during liposuction or if an open

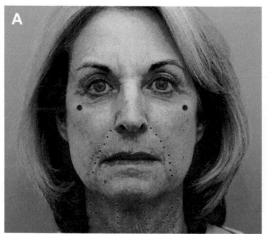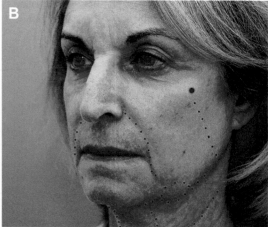

Fig. 3. (*A* and *B*) Preoperative facial markings with patient in upright position.

platysmal tightening procedure is planned. A 2-0 silk tie is wrapped and tied around each of the two central incisors and then around the endotracheal tube. If teeth are missing, a 2-0 silk suture is placed in the gingivo-buccal sulcus through the periosteum and tied to the endotracheal tube. To prevent excessive pulling on the tube with head turning during surgery, a rubber "accordion" extension is placed at the end of the endotracheal tube. This extension provides additional slack for the circuit and enables easier and safer head repositioning during the procedure. When prepping the patient and the endotracheal tube, the authors prefer to keep the tube exposed throughout the case, so no untoward events occur during changes in head positioning. This exposure is accomplished by prepping the proximal segment of the tube with Betadine and wrapping the distal segment with sterile blue towels. Some surgeons prefer to use clear sticky drapes on the tube, but the authors have found this method to be complex and unnecessary; in some cases sticky drapes interfere with adjustments of the endotracheal tube during the surgery. Next, the patient's body is pulled up to the top of the headrest. Such positioning is essential for establishing easier access to submental structures. All pressure points (elbows, knees, and heels) are reviewed with a circulating nurse and are padded adequately with egg crate foam (elbows and heels) and pillows (knees).

Instrumentation

Whether operating at a hospital, an outpatient surgery center, or in one's private office, it is critical to select personally the instruments for the rhytidectomy tray. The authors have found that surgical sets from high-volume operating rooms often contain blunt instruments, making precise and delicate surgical maneuvers more difficult than need be. When operating at a hospital, the authors bring the critical instruments with them to help prevent interruptions to the flow of surgery.

The authors have found several instruments to be particularly useful during facelift surgery. Facelift scissors come in all shapes and sizes, and the surgeon must be comfortable and familiar with this instrument. The authors have found supercut scissors manufactured by Accurate Surgical & Scientific Instruments (Westbury, New York) to be particularly helpful. The supercut blades are extremely sharp and cut skin much like a scalpel. They are available in a large variety of shapes and sizes, are extremely durable, are not particularly costly, and have excellent customer service support. The particular models the authors prefer are the Kaye-Freeman 18-cm curved with spread shanks, tapered tips, and serrated blades (**Fig. 4**A). They are ergonomically designed, extremely sharp, and easy to use in flap undermining and dissection. Other scissor models from this vendor include the 14-cm curved Joseph and 17-cm curved Matarasso (**Fig. 4**B). Instruments useful in flap retraction include the Millard thimble hook, 1-inch-wide double-prong skin hooks, Freeman rake, Anderson bear claw, and the Converse nasal retractor. For open platysmal procedures, a fiberoptic lighted submental retractor is particularly helpful and frees the surgeon from wearing a cumbersome headlight.

Incisions

Before incisions are designed, a proper marking pen is required. Many markers are too thick or coarse, whereas very fine-tipped pens with delicate tips (which are good for eyelid surgery

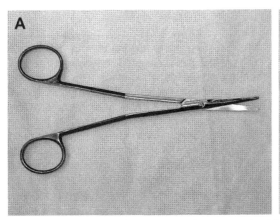
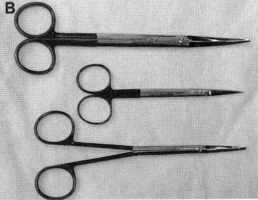

Fig. 4. (*A*) Kaye-Freeman facelift scissor (Accurate Scientific and Surgical Instruments Corporation, New York, New York). (*B*) Standard facelift scissors (Accurate Scientific and Surgical Instruments Corporation, New York, New York).

markings) are too fine for facial procedures and can run out of ink too quickly. The authors prefer a marking pen manufactured by Aspen Surgical (Caledonia, Michigan) that has the benefits of both a fine and a thicker tip (**Fig. 5**).

A facelift incision is marked around the auricle. Several important concepts guide the placement of the periauricular incision, which forms the initial measure for avoiding several dreaded complications of face lifting, such as temporal wasting, tragal eversion, pixie ear deformity, and posterior hairline step-offs.

In patients who have a high temporal tuft or excessive temporal laxity, the authors modify the temporal portion of the incision with a sideburn extension (**Fig. 6**). This modification creates a superiorly based temporal advancement-rotation flap that preserves temporal hair and keeps the temporal hairline down. Incision marking in front of the auricle follows the curvature of the helical root, passes over the tragal top in women (in front of the tragus in men), and curves around the lobule into the postauricular crease. In short-scar facelifts this incision stops just at the level of the external auditory canal, but in more traditional procedures the postauricular component of the incision connects to the hairline at the auricular–hairline junction and darts posteriorly at the level of the tragus.

After the markings, the hair is parted with a comb along incision lines and is bound with small rubber bands. Wetting hair with a lubricating ointment, such as Surgilube or Bacitracin, greatly assists in this process. The face then is prepped with Betadine and is draped with full face and neck exposure.

Within hair-bearing regions (temporal and posterior), incisions are appropriately beveled to

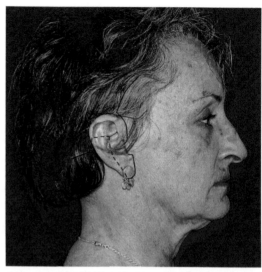

Fig. 6. Facelift incisions. See text for detailed description. Curved red line indicates a sideburn incision, used to control the extent of temporal hairline elevation.

preserve hair follicles and avoid postoperative alopecia. The angulation of hair shafts at these sites can be especially acute, forming a 10° to 20° angle with respect to the plane of the scalp. The surgeon should avoid making a full-thickness incision in one move and instead should perform several strokes while visualizing and following hair shafts at all times. This technique allows maximal preservation of hair follicles at incision sites. In addition, monopolar and bipolar electrocautery should be used judiciously around bleeding scalp edges, because it may induce thermal injury to hair follicles. Persistently oozy skin edges can be controlled effectively by a local anesthetic injection with 1% lidocaine and 1:100,000 units of epinephrine.

Dissection

After initial incisions are made with a fresh #15 blade, a skin flap is elevated under direct visualization in the subcutaneous plane. The surgeon can develop this dissection easily and quickly with the assistance of a thimble hook retractor. Overhead lights are positioned directly over the face, transilluminating the skin flap and aiding in maintaining a uniform surgical plane Once this plane is further developed anteriorly, the straight end of a Converse retractor can be used easily to move freely under the flap. In the authors' experience, bleeding on the undersurface of the skin flap is controlled best with unipolar cautery, which causes far fewer skin burns than a bipolar instrument. In contrast, deeper bleeding tissues are

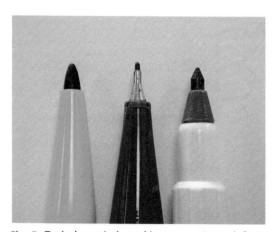

Fig. 5. Typical surgical marking pens. From left to right: regular tip, very fine tip, combination tip (Aspen Surgical, Caledonia, Michigan).

coagulated more effectively and safely with bipolar cautery. The extent of subcutaneous dissection depends in large part on the surgical technique and clinical presentation of the patient. In nonsmokers with heavy jowls, a long skin flap elevated anteriorly over the jowl is especially useful in providing access for direct trimming of the jowl. For those undergoing a deep-plane face-lift, a shorter subcutaneous dissection is performed. In standard lateral superficial muscular aponeurotic system (SMAS) techniques, the sub-SMAS dissection begins by identifying the pre-parotid plane anterior to the auricle. A J-shaped segment of SMAS can be excised safely with face-lift scissors at this location. Anteriorly, proper identification of a sub-SMAS plane can be assisted by hydrodissecting with several cubic centimeters of saline solution. In most instances, release of parotid-cutaneous and masseteric-cutaneous retaining ligaments provides the necessary mobilization of the deep facial plane.

Closure

Only two relative tension points are created during skin closure, with both affixed to deep fascia to ensure long-term stabilization of the skin flap. In the temporal region, immediately superior to the auricle, the skin flap is placed on gentle stretch in the postero-superior direction. Care is taken to avoid overpulling (creating a wind-blown appearance and temporal wasting) or extreme superior pull (creating temporal bunching). A half-mattress suture is placed through the skin edges as well as deep temporal fascia to achieve fixation at this anatomic location. Posterior to the auricle, the direction of pull is essentially superior, ensuring proper alignment of the occipital hairline and avoiding step-offs. A half-mattress suture is placed similarly in this location, incorporating the mastoid periosteum.

The remainder of skin closure is performed tension-free to avoid developing tell-tale signs of facelifting, such as anteriorly pulled tragus and satyr ear. To achieve this closure, facial flap skin is trimmed precisely around the periphery of the auricle so that no tension is required during closure. The pretragal sulcus is recreated by thinning pretragal skin to the level of the dermis and placing a 4-0 Vicryl suture from dermis to the perichondrium of the medial tragus. Skin at the ear lobule is closed while incorporating the lobular ligament. All incisions in the occipital and temporal hair-bearing regions are closed with staples. The remainder of skin is closed with a simple running 6-0 nylon suture. After skin closure, all incisions are washed with saline and half-strength peroxide.

Drains and Dressings

The single most important measure to prevent post-operative hematoma is meticulous intraoperative hemostasis. When drains are used, flat size #10 Jackson-Pratt (JP) drains are placed on each side and are passed through separate stab incisions within hair-bearing scalp. No sutures are used because the drains are held firmly in place by the neck of JP and are removed on the first postoperative day. Bacitracin ointment is applied liberally over incision sites, and Telfa pads are placed around the ears. A light pressure dressing consisting of fluffs and a 3-inch Kling flexible dressing (Johnson & Johnson, Langhorne, Pennsylvania) is applied around the neck and face. Fishnet stockinet material is quick and easy to use and keeps the dressing in place. Simply stretch the stockinet over the entire head and tear a whole for the face while tying a knot in the top to prevent slippage. Alternately, a 3-inch Coban dressing (3M Healthcare, St. Paul, Minnesota) can be used. With Coban, one can regulate the amount of compression support while providing an aesthetically acceptable, skin-colored dressing that prevents slippage.

POSTOPERATIVE PEARLS
Postoperative Day #1

On the first postoperative day, the surgical dressing is removed, and the face and neck are inspected for bruising, ischemia, and collections. Because this visit may occur in a hospital, an overnight facility, or even the patient's home, all the supplies required for this dressing change are brought along. Small collections can be drained easily with a medium-bore (21-gauge to 25-gauge) needle. Local anesthetic is not required for this percutaneous drainage, because the skin is sufficiently anesthetized from the facelift dissection. Large or recurrent collections can be treated by inserting an Angiocath (14 gauge or 16 gauge) and leaving it in place with a pressure dressing for a couple of days. Placement of an Angiocath allows continuing drainage and hastens the adherence of skin to the underlying tissues.

Patients are instructed to ice for the first 48 to 72 hours, to sleep on several pillows, and to avoid strenuous activity. They may advance their diet as tolerated and begin taking their usual medications. They should not drive or make important decisions while taking narcotics or sedatives in the immediate postoperative period. Patients are given a facial compression garment and are instructed to wear it around the clock for the first week. This frequency changes to nightly use after 1 week. Patients should be

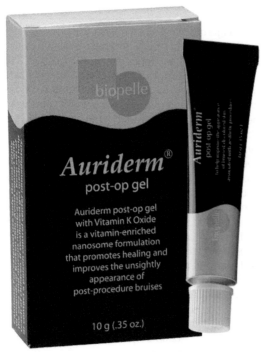

Fig. 7. Auriderm postoperative gel. (Photograph courtesy of Biopelle, Ferndale, Michigan; with permission.)

taking their regimen of *Arnica Montana*, bromelain, and antibiotics.

Postoperative Day #3

Patients may begin showering and gently shampooing their hair. They are instructed to massage their scalp gently, rinse with tepid water, and avoid hair-coloring products for several weeks. This wound-care regimen is important in keeping incisions clear of crusting, which greatly assists with suture removal. Ecchymosis is diminished further with twice-daily application of Auriderm postoperative gel (Biopelle, Ferndale, Michigan) with vitamin K oxide (**Fig. 7**).

Patients may gradually increase their routine daily activities at this point while avoiding bending, lifting, and other strenuous activity. Light exercise

may commence after 3 weeks, depending on individual progress and recovery.

Postoperative Day #7

All sutures and staples are removed at this point, and wounds are inspected. Areas of significant bruising or palpable firmness can be treated with several sessions of ultrasound shock-wave therapy (RICH-MAR 510, Byron Medical, Tucson, Arizona). Patients are instructed to massage gently any areas of firmness and to use heat pads as necessary.

Postoperative Weeks #1 to 4

Hypertrophic and erythematous surgical scars respond well to topical silicone gel therapy. The authors prefer Scarguard gel (Scarguard Labs, Great Neck, New York), which comes with its own application brush, making it easily to apply around facelift incisions. More extreme measures include pulsed dye laser therapy,[4] which can be given several times a few weeks apart. For thickened scars, conservative steroid injections (Kenalog 10, Bristol-Myers, Princeton, New Jersey) can be initiated for any subcutaneous irregularities. A routine follow-up sequence consists of office visits at 3, 6, and 12 months and annually thereafter.

REFERENCES

1. Seeley BM, Denton AB, Ahn MS, et al. Effect of homeopathic Arnica Montana on bruising in face-lifts: results of a randomized, double-blind, placebo-controlled clinical trial. Arch Facial Plast Surg 2006;8(1):54–9.
2. Orsini RA. Bromelain. Plast Reconstr Surg 2006; 118(7):1640–4.
3. Maurer HR. Bromelain: biochemistry, pharmacology and medical use. Cell Mol Life Sci 2001;58(9):1234–45.
4. Nouri K, Jimenez GP, Harrison-Balestra C, et al. 585-nm pulsed dye laser in the treatment of surgical scars starting on the suture removal day. Dermatol Surg 2003;29(1):65–73.

Discussion Regarding Botulinum Toxin, Immunologic Considerations with Long-term Repeated Use, with Emphasis on Cosmetic Applications

Article by Gary Borodic, MD, Published in February 2007 Facial Plastic Surgery Clinics

MINIMAL RISK OF ANTIBODY FORMATION AFTER AESTHETIC TREATMENT WITH TYPE A BOTULINUM TOXIN

Andy Pickett, PhD[a,*], David Caird, PhD[b]

The article by Dr Borodic,[1] on immunological considerations for the long-term use of botulinum toxin A in aesthetic medicine, raises a number of interesting issues. However, one important point that must be borne in mind, in any such discussion, is that the total protein content of the product being administered (toxin complexes with various protective non-toxin proteins) is not relevant for the production of neutralizing antibodies (NAb) to the toxin. The original Botox formulation, produced from bulk toxin batch 79–11 as provided by Dr Schantz in Wisconsin, contained about 90% inactivated toxin due to both the age of the material and the salt precipitation and lyophilization method used for final product preparation.[2] This product correspondingly had a higher immunogenic potential than one without the inactivated toxin. Changing the bulk toxin batch used in this formulation reduced the immune challenge and, consequently, the rate of NAb formation.[3,4]

The protective protein complex itself is not believed to be relevant for the production of NAb to the neurotoxin molecule. The complex is pH sensitive and rapidly dissociates under physiological conditions, releasing the neurotoxin molecule. This sensitivity has been described in Schantz and Johnson's classic review papers[5–7] as a means of obtaining pure toxin. In vitro experiments have shown this dissociation to be both complete and rapid.[8] Any antibodies to other proteins in the complex will not be NAb; any Western blot or other analytical test that cannot distinguish between these other antibodies and NAb is not clinically useful.[9–11] Currently, no in vitro method can distinguish this difference. Therefore, in vivo or ex vivo tests must be used, such as the mouse protection assay (MPA) and the mouse phrenic hemidiaphragm assay (MPHA).[9] Alternatively, pragmatic tests on patient wrinkles,[1] the extensor digitorum brevis muscle,[12] or sweat glands[13] have been used by clinicians but are only applicable to the individuals concerned and are not suitable for screening or epidemiological studies.

In contrast to Dr Borodic's view,[1] the authors have found the MPA to be very sensitive for the assessment of patient sera, the method being routinely capable of determining the neutralization of 1 median lethal dose (LD_{50}) unit of type A toxin (equivalent to 0.0001 units/mL of type A botulinum antitoxin) or lower.[9] The MPHA is able to detect NAb titers to a sensitivity of 0.0003 units antitoxin/mL,[10] which is, in turn, approximately 30 to 300 times more sensitive than in vitro methods such as an ELISA assay.[10,11]

Dr Borodic states that there are no long-term studies of NAb formation in patients treated for facial wrinkles. However, there is a considerable body of relevant data from indications using significantly higher doses of the two main commercial preparations, Dysport and Botox. These are especially relevant when considering the overall rate of antibody formation to toxin treatment. In Germany, two long-term studies have been carried out with

---

Gary Borodic is a consultant for Mentor Corporation (a Johnson and Johnson Company).

[a] Biologicals Science and Technology, Ash Road, Ipsen Biopharm Limited, Wrexham LL139UF, UK
[b] Ipsen Pharma GmbH, Einsteinstrasse 30, Ettlingen D-76275, Germany
* Corresponding author.
E-mail address: andy.pickett@ipsen.com (A. Pickett).

Facial Plast Surg Clin N Am 17 (2009) 633–637
doi:10.1016/j.fsc.2009.07.003

Dysport, which has been marketed in the same formulation since 1990: one vial of Dysport contains 500 Ipsen mouse LD_{50} units of toxin in 4.35 ng of protein complex.[5] An earlier study reported data from 303 patients with cervical dystonia (CD) treated for a mean of 3.2 years (mean 10.2 treatments), of whom 17 showed secondary nonresponse, and 9 (3%) were NAb-positive according to the MPHA.[14] NAb formation was significantly correlated with so-called booster injections at short intervals in this early 1999 study. Booster injections are no longer carried out, for this very reason. A 2004 study on 100 CD patients, treated with Dysport for a mean of 5.1 years and including a subgroup of 32 patients treated for a mean of 10 years in one clinic, identified just three secondary nonresponse patients, none of whom showed NAb in the MPHA test.[15]

Long-term data in high dose indications for patients treated only with the present formulation of Botox, introduced around 1998, are available. In post-stroke spasticity (111 patients treated for a mean period of 54 weeks) and CD (326 patients with a median of 9 treatments), NAb were detected in 0.6% and 1.23% of patients respectively, using the MPA.[16,17]

Taken together, these data suggest that the risk of NAb formation, even after several years of use at high therapeutic doses, is low with either Dysport or the present formulation of Botox, at least in adults. The corresponding risk in low-dose use for the treatment of wrinkles must be significantly reduced. The case reported by Dr Borodic[1,18] is, to our knowledge, the only one in the literature—despite the fact that injections of botulinum toxin type A to treat facial wrinkles are now the most common procedure in aesthetic medicine.[19] Also, the published long-term data on the aesthetic use of Dysport[20] and Botox[21,22] do not suggest any cause for concern. Dr Borodic is correct to draw attention to the potential consequences of NAb formation due to the use of botulinum toxin type A in aesthetic medicine, but the risk of this happening appears to be very low.

RESPONSE RELATIVE TO PHARMACEUTICAL COMPOSITION OF BOTULINUM TOXIN FOR HUMAN INJECTION, CLINICAL EXPERIENCE WITH INCIDENCE OF ANTIBODY FORMATION, THE ACTUAL ANTIBODY TESTS, AND SOME ETHICAL CONSIDERATIONS REGARDING THE EVOLVING USES AS A THERAPEUTIC AND COSMETIC PHARMACEUTICAL

Gary Borodic, MD
e-mail: borodic@aol.com

As Dr Pickett states, the composition of the 79-11 batch of botulinum toxin used in the United States between 1983 and 1998 did contain a much higher protein content and correspondingly low specific activity. This preparation contained between about 40 ng per 100 U vial (specific activity 2.5 u/ng).[1,2] The large amount of toxin based protein in the vials included:

1. Active neurotoxin (active ingredient)
2. Inactivated neurotoxin from stored source materials or formulation deterioration during lyophilization
3. Adjuvant "complex" proteins (hemagglutinin, non-hemagglutinin–non-neurotoxin proteins).

The large inactivated neurotoxin protein component of the original formulation was the major concern, as deactivated neurotoxin still can have immunogenic properties.[1,3,4] As considerable amounts of both inactive neurotoxin protein was present in earlier formulations, the incidence of antibody production with secondary resistance was 17% in higher-dose cervical dystonia studies using the mouse-neutralizing detection method over a period of 3 to 5 years.[5] Lower-dose indications receiving lower neurotoxin protein load per injections cycle were associated much less commonly with antibody formation.[1] The differences in the rate of neutralizing antibody development between high dose indications such as cervical dystonia (higher neurotoxin protein exposures per injection) and low-dose indications such as hemifacial spasm and blepharospasm (lower neurotoxin protein exposure per injection cycle) provided motivation to reduce the neurotoxin protein per vial, which was accomplished in the botulinum type A toxin (BOTOX) product in 1998.[6] The originators of botulinum toxin manufacturing at the University of Wisconsin were concerned about the quality of neurotoxin in the early BOTOX-Oculinum preparations.[2,7,8]

Since 1998, the commercially available type A botulinum toxin complex in the United States, BOTOX, was modified by its commercial manufacturer to a much higher specific activity with attendant reduction in total protein to approximately 5 ng per 100 U vial. As Dr Pickett has accurately pointed out, this formulation change clearly reduced, but did not eliminate, the incidence of secondary resistance.[9-11] The impact of the formulation change on reduction of antibody formation rate was most notable for cervical dystonia,[9] the prototype high-dose long-term botulinum toxin indication. From these observations, study results, and experience, the most ideal formulation of botulinum toxin for human use is one in which the amount of neurotoxin protein in vials is minimized, eliminating as much inactive and unnecessary neurotoxin as possible, while maintaining a high clinical potency per unit activity dosage.[1] The changes in the BOTOX formulation in 1998 were an initial and effective step in this direction.

Clinically significant "neutralizing" antibodies to botulinum toxin are conventionally measured with a mouse protection assay which uses a fixed amount of patient's serum, a lethal dose of botulinum toxin to the reference mouse, and the recipient mice who either survive (positive assay) or are killed by injections of the mixture within 3 to 4 days (negative assay). This assay was originally designed to measure effectiveness of botulinum toxoids (vaccines) with respect to conferring immunity. In this application, the sera of scientist's immunized with botulinum toxoid originally testing positive can drop significantly, indicating the need for booster vaccinations. From the physician and surgeons' perspective, there are also problems with this assay. Patients who have developed secondary resistance achieving no weakness in targeted or remote point muscles may be negative to this assay. Even patients with well-documented resistance originally positive to neutralizing mouse assay can show negative results over time. For this reason, the remote point clinical testing for weakness became popular over the last 15 years.[12–14] Patients testing negative for mouse neutralizing antibodies can have positive remote point tests. From a physiologic perspective, the mouse assay also may lack correlation to tissue pharmacokinetics. When the surgeon injects botulinum toxin into a muscle, the toxin becomes *in transient,* binding to presynaptic membrane receptors, internalization, ultimately reacting with the cytoplasmic substrate. During this transient time before receptor mediated internalization, the molecule is vulnerable to antitoxin (from hours to about 1–2 days).[15] The interstitial fluid perfusing the muscle may be much greater than the amount gathered within small-volume serum specimen used in the mouse bioassay. The serum volume concentration multiple may be the reason for the strong predictive value and possible higher sensitivity of the remote point type tests than the mouse assay. This tissue kinetic may explain the higher confidence in remote point "individual" assessment tests referred to by Dr Pickett and colleagues.

Regional hindlimb paralysis assays and tissue bath nerve-muscle preparation may suffer some of the same criticisms, although they probably have a small increased toxin sensitivity over the mouse assay. As neutralizing antibodies may differ in quantity and binding affinities to the neurotoxin, low-level or low-affinity antibodies in the test tube with a small sera specimen may still be clinically significant. Newer in vitro assays that demonstrate the highest toxin sensitivity system may offer the best chance for a more sensitive in vitro antibody test. In this respect, the cultured neuronal cell assay, which detects both botulinum toxin membrane receptor binding and cytoplasmic substrate-SNAP 25 cleavage, is under evaluation and may offer an improved method of assay. The assay has been reported to have a toxin sensitivity to 0.1 U,[16] about 10 X that of the mouse detection assay sensitivity in the mouse detection system referred to by Dr Pickett.

Appropriately, the major supplier of BOTOX has made it clear on the package insert that long-term studies in the cosmetic use of botulinum toxin are lacking.[5] Many patients using botulinum toxin for cosmetic purposes do so for many years and many will receive ongoing injections over a period of decades going forward. For many, the treatment is a lifelong endeavor. Secondary immunity in the past has usually required a number of years to develop (usually 3–6 years for cervical dystonia). Studies involving 3 to 9 injection cycles may not be adequate exposure paradigms to make any firm conclusions, particularly in light of a low-sensitivity mouse assay. From a clinical perspective, the cosmetic patient who may become immune may be less likely to report the secondary resistance because they judge the injections as ineffective and become "lost to follow-up." In contrast, the therapeutic patient would continue to suffer and to seek relief from chronic disease. Since publication of the original articles, I have still another cosmetic case demonstrating both neutralizing antibodies to the mouse assay and neuronal cell assay. In my practice, a fraction of the patient population with neurologic blepharospasm who has received repeated injections for 1 to 2 decades relate a reduced response over time, without clear explanation. These patients often receive the same dose range as the cosmetic population. Other physicians have noted secondary resistance even with lower doses of the newer preparations.[17]

Wide-scale use of the toxin as a cosmetic will probably lead to many cosmetic recipients needing future therapeutic injections if they develop stroke, spasticity, prostatic hypertrophy, certain headaches, or many of the other therapeutic indications known to be responsive to toxin technology. Although it is clear that the risk in the short term is small, the long term is still unknown.

Given the weaknesses inherent in current assay techniques, the cross-usage of the medication, the higher standard of safety inherently needed for cosmetic applications for acceptable risk–benefit assessments, the need for accurate informed consent, further assay development, knowledge of compositional pharmacology, and clinical study—assessment of antibody formation rates are needed for the cosmetic patient, as has been conducted for other indications.

As Dr Pickett and colleagues have brought up the issue regarding fractional inactivation and denaturation of botulinum toxin production during lyophilization in the original 79-11 preparation, it would be helpful if manufacturers revealed percent biologic-activity loss during drying and preparation process. Creation of inactive and potentially immunogenic neurotoxin can occur during this step of the process, as Dr Pickett has pointed out. The loss of biologic activity during the drying process indicates the conversion of active neurotoxin to inactive neurotoxin. Drying recovery data may be useful in comparing preparations of the same immunotype for purity that has been linked to immunogenicity. Additionally, each manufacturer should reveal the total protein quantity and compositions in the vials inclusive of an estimated mass of botulinum neurotoxin, complexing proteins (if present), method of LD 50 bioassay, gel protein electrophoresis, and albumin concentrations so that the many clinicians using these materials can better understand and evaluate the differences between available preparations from a pharmacologic perspective, and make their own judgments.

REFERENCES: PICKETT AND CAIRD DISCUSSION: MINIMAL RISK OF ANTIBODY FORMATION AFTER AESTHETIC TREATMENT WITH TYPE A BOTULINUM TOXININ

1. Borodic G. Botulinum toxin, immunologic considerations with long-term repeated use, with emphasis on cosmetic applications. Facial Plast Surg Clin North Am 2007;15:11–6.
2. Goodnough MC, Johnson EA. Stabilization of botulinum toxin type A during lyophilization. Appl Environ Microbiol 1992;58:3426–8.
3. Aoki K. Preclinical update on Botox (botulinum toxin type A)-purified neurotoxin complex relative to other botulinum neurotoxin preparations. Eur J Neurol 1999;6(Suppl 4):S3–S10.
4. Jankovic J, Vuong KD, Ahsan J. Comparison of efficacy and immunogenicity of original versus current botulinum toxin in cervical dystonia. Neurology 2003;60:1186–8.
5. Pickett AM, O'Keefe R, Panjwani N. The protein load of therapeutic botulinum toxins. Eur J Neurol 2007; 14:e11.
6. Schantz EJ, Johnson EA. Properties and use of botulinum toxin and other microbial neurotoxins in medicine. Microbiol Rev 1992;56:80–99.
7. Schantz EJ, Johnson EA. Botulinum toxin: the story of its development for the treatment of human disease. Perspect Biol Med 1997;40:317–27.
8. Friday D, Bigalke H, Frevert J. In vitro stability of botulinum toxin complex preparations at physiological pH and temperature. Naunyn Schmiedebergs Arch Pharmacol 2002;365(Suppl 2):R20.
9. Duane DD, Pickett AM. Assessment of antibody development in patients treated with type A botulinum toxin, presented at the Third International Dystonia Symposium. Miami, FL. Oct 11, 1996.
10. Goschel H, Wohlfarth K, Frevert J, et al. Botulinum A toxin therapy: neutralizing and nonneutralizing antibodies—therapeutic consequences. Exp Neurol 1997;147:96–102.
11. Sesardic D, Jones RG, Leung T, et al. Detection of antibodies against botulinum toxins. Mov Disord 2004;19(Suppl 8):S85–91.
12. Kessler KR, Benecke R. The EBD test—a clinical test for the detection of antibodies to botulinum toxin type A. Mov Disord 1997;12(1):95–9.
13. Voller B, Moraru E, Auff E, et al. Ninhydrin sweat test: a simple method for detecting antibodies neutralizing botulinum toxin type A. Mov Disord 2004 Aug;19(8):943–7.
14. Kessler KR, Skutta M, Benecke R. Long-term treatment of cervical dystonia with botulinum toxin A: efficacy, safety, and antibody frequency. German Dystonia Study Group. J Neurol 1999;246:265–74.
15. Haussermann P, Marczoch S, Klinger C, et al. Long-term follow-up of cervical dystonia patients treated with botulinum toxin A. Mov Disord 2004;19:303–8.
16. Turkel C, Dru R, Dagget S, et al. Neutralizing antibody formation is rare following repeated injections of a low protein formulation of botulinum toxin type A in patients with post-stroke spasticity. Neurology 2002;58(Suppl 3):A316.
17. Yablon S, Dagget S, Lai F, et al. The development of toxin neutralizing antibodies with botulinum toxin type A (BoNTA) treatment. Neurorehabil Neural Repair 2006;20:176–7.
18. Borodic G. Immunologic resistance after repeated botulinum toxin type A injections for facial rhytides. Ophthal Plast Reconstr Surg 2006;22:239–40.
19. Klein AW. The clinical use of botulinum toxin. Dermatol Clin 2004;22:ix.
20. Rzany B, Dill-Muller D, Grablowitz D, et al. Repeated botulinum toxin A injections for the treatment of lines in the upper face: a retrospective study of 4,103 treatments in 945 patients. Dermatol Surg 2007; 33(Suppl 1):S18–25.

21. Bulstrode NW, Grobbelaar AO. Long-term prospective follow-up of botulinum toxin treatment for facial rhytides. Aesthetic Plast Surg 2002;26:356–9.

22. Carruthers A, Carruthers J. Long-term safety review of subjects treated with botulinum toxin type A (BoNT/A) for cosmetic use. From the 5th International Conference on Basic and Therapeutic Aspects of Botulinum and Tetanus Toxins, 23–25 June 2005, Denver, CO, USA. p. P03.

REFERENCES: BORODIC DISCUSSION: BOTOX FOR HUMAN INJECTION, CLINICAL EXPERIENCE WITH ANTIBODY FORMATION

1. Borodic G, Johnson E, Goodnough M, et al. Botulinum toxin, immunologic resistance and problems with available materials. Neurology 1996;46:26–9.

2. Goodnough MC, Johnson EA. Stabilization of botulinum toxin type A during lyophilization. Appl Environ Microbiol 1992;58:3426–8.

3. Schantz EJ, Johnson EA. Properties and use of botulinum toxin and other microbial neurotoxins in medicine. Microbiol Rev 1992;56:80–99.

4. Schantz EJ, Johnson EA. Botulinum toxin: the story of its development for the treatment of human disease. Perspect Biol Med 1997;40:317–27.

5. Package Insert for BOTOX, Allergan Pharmaceuticals.

6. Allergan Announcement – Maintaining Response to botulinum toxin therapy, 1999.

7. Schantz E. Introduction textbook of botulinum toxin therapy. In: Jankovic J, Hallet M, editors. Therapy with botulinum toxin. New York, Hong Kong: Marcel Dekker; 1994. p. 23–7.

8. Schantz E, Johnson E. Characterization of botulinum toxin type A for human treatment textbook of botulinum toxin therapy. In: Jankovic J, Hallet M, editors. Therapy with botulinum toxin. New York, Hong Kong: Marcel Dekker; 1994. p. 41–51.

9. Jankovic J, Vuong KD, Ahsan J. Comparison of efficacy and immunogenicity of original versus current botulinum toxin in cervical dystonia. Neurology 2003;60:1186–8.

10. Kessler KR, Skutta M, Benecke R. Long-term treatment of cervical dystonia with botulinum toxin A: efficacy, safety, and antibody frequency. German Dystonia Study Group. J Neurol 1999;246:265–74.

11. Kessler KR, Benecke R. The EBD test—a clinical test for the detection of antibodies to botulinum toxin type A. Mov Disord 1997;12(1):95–9.

12. Borodic GE. Botulinum toxin issues and applications. Curr Opin Otolaryngol Head Neck Surg 1999;352(9143):1832.

13. Borodic GE, Pearce LB, Duane D, et al. Antibodies to botulinum toxin. Neurology 1995;45(1):204.

14. Hanna PA, Jankovic J, Vincent A. Comparison of mouse bioassay and immunoprecipitation assay for botulinum toxin antibodies. J Neurol Neurosurg Psychiatr 1999;66(5):612–6.

15. Mayer CN, Holley JL, Brooks T. Antitoxin therapy for botulinum intoxication. Rev Med Micro 2001;12:29–37.

16. Pellett S, Tepp WH, Clancy CM, et al. A neuronal cell-based botulinum neurotoxin assay for highly sensitive and specific detection of neutralizing serum antibodies. FEBS Lett 2007;581(25):4803–8.

17. Dressler D. New formulation of BOTOX, complete antibody therapy induced failure in hemifacial spasm. J Neurol 2004;251(3):360.

Index

Note: Page numbers of article titles are in **boldface** type

A

Ablative fractional laser resurfacing, as facelift adjunct, 513

Adjunctive techniques, for facelifts, **505–514**
alloplastic augmentation as, 511
laser lipolysis-assisted contouring as, basic steps of, 507–508
of jawline, 511
of melolabial fold, 506–510
of lower facial third, 508, 511
of middle facial third, 505–506
skin rejuvenation as, 512–513
submalar augmentation as, 506
summary overview of, 505, 514
for neck rejuvenation, 598–600
botulinum toxin type A as, 599–600
fat grafting as, 599
LAL as, 599–600

Aesthetic facial surgery, adjunctive techniques for, **505–514**. See also *Adjunctive techniques.*
ASA risk-assessment classification system for, 532
botulinum toxin vs., **633–637**. See also *Botulinum toxin A.*
consultation for. See *Consultation.*
facelifts as. See *Facelifts.*
heavy neck and, **603–611**. See also *Heavy neck.*
in men, **613–624**
avoiding facelift complications and, 622–623
consultation for, 614–615
decision making factors of, 615–616, 618
demographic trends in, 614
dichotomous sentiment examples of, 616–621
dissatisfied patients and, 623–624
effective communication and management process for, 614–615, 623–624
long-term follow-up of, 623
patient education on, 618–619
perioperative considerations of, 619–622
postoperative care of, 618–619, 624
summary overview of, 613, 624
vs. women, 613–614

Age/aging, facial, in preoperative evaluation, for facelifts, 516
process of, in lower facial third, 508–511, 589–590
in neck, 589–590
volumetric facelift and, 539–541

Airway management, during anesthesia, for facelifts, 533–534
intraoperative pearls for, 628–629

Alloplastic augmentation, as facelift adjunct, 511

American Society of Anesthesiologists (ASA), risk-assessment classification system of, for elective cosmetic surgical patients, 532

Anchor sutures, for short-scar purse-string facelift, 553–556

Anesthesia management, for facelifts, **531–538**
airway considerations, 533–534
intraoperative pearls for, 628–629
hypertension and, 536
induction, intraoperative, 628–629
inhalational anesthetics, 535–536
intravenous anesthetics, 536
intravenous sedation, 537–538
local anesthetics, 533–535. See also *Local anesthetics.*
bupivacaine as, 535
cocaine as, 535
lidocaine as, 535
mechanism of action, 534–535
mixed solutions, 533–534
nausea and, 536–537
patient safety and, 532–534
preoperative preparation and screening, 531–532
summary overview of, 531, 538

Anesthetics, inhalational, for facelifts, 535–536
intravenous, for facelifts, 536
local, for facelifts, 533–535. See also *Local anesthetics.*

Antibiotics, postoperative, for facelifts, 632

Antibody formation, with botulinum toxin A injections, actual tests for, 635
clinical incidence of, 634–635
long-term studies on, 635
minimal risk of, 633–634

Aprepitant (Emend), for postoperative nausea prevention, with facelifts, 537

Arnica Montana, for facelifts, 627, 632

Augmentation procedures, as facelift adjunct, alloplastic, 511
midface, 505–506
submalar, 506

Auricular deformities, with facelifts, 520, 620

Auricular incisions, for extended superficial musculoaponeurotic system rhytidectomy, 580–584
for facelifts, intraoperative markings for, 630
for neck rejuvenation, 596, 598

Auriderm postoperative gel, for facelifts, 632

Facial Plast Surg Clin N Am 17 (2009) 639–648
doi:10.1016/S1064-7406(09)00118-7
1064-7406/09/$ – see front matter © 2009 Elsevier Inc. All rights reserved.

facialplastic.theclinics.com

United States Postal Service

Statement of Ownership, Management, and Circulation
(All Periodicals Publications Except Requestor Publications)

1. Publication Title	2. Publication Number	3. Filing Date
Facial Plastic Surgery Clinics of North America	0 1 1 3 - 1 2 2 2	9/15/09

4. Issue Frequency	5. Number of Issues Published Annually	6. Annual Subscription Price
Feb, May, Aug, Nov	4	$273.00

7. Complete Mailing Address of Known Office of Publication (Not printer) (Street, city, county, state, and ZIP+4®)

Elsevier Inc.
360 Park Avenue South
New York, NY 10010-1710

Contact Person
Stephen Bushing

Telephone (Include area code)
215-239-3688

8. Complete Mailing Address of Headquarters or General Business Office of Publisher (Not printer)

Elsevier Inc., 360 Park Avenue South, New York, NY 10010-1710

9. Full Names and Complete Mailing Addresses of Publisher, Editor, and Managing Editor (Do not leave blank)

Publisher (Name and complete mailing address)

John Schrefer, Elsevier, Inc., 1600 John F. Kennedy Blvd. Suite 1800, Philadelphia, PA 19103-2899

Editor (Name and complete mailing address)

Joanne Husovski, Elsevier, Inc., 1600 John F. Kennedy Blvd. Suite 1800, Philadelphia, PA 19103-2899

Managing Editor (Name and complete mailing address)

Catherine Bewick, Elsevier, Inc., 1600 John F. Kennedy Blvd. Suite 1800, Philadelphia, PA 19103-2899

10. Owner (Do not leave blank. If the publication is owned by a corporation, give the name and address of the corporation immediately followed by the names and addresses of all stockholders owning or holding 1 percent or more of the total amount of stock. If not owned by a corporation, give the names and addresses of the individual owners. If owned by a partnership or other unincorporated firm, give its name and address as well as those of each individual owner. If the publication is published by a nonprofit organization, give its name and address.)

Full Name	Complete Mailing Address
Wholly owned subsidiary of	4520 East-West Highway
Reed/Elsevier, US holdings	Bethesda, MD 20814

11. Known Bondholders, Mortgagees, and Other Security Holders Owning or Holding 1 Percent or More of Total Amount of Bonds, Mortgages, or Other Securities. If none, check box ☐ None

Full Name	Complete Mailing Address
N/A	

12. Tax Status (For completion by nonprofit organizations authorized to mail at nonprofit rates) (Check one)
The purpose, function, and nonprofit status of this organization and the exempt status for federal income tax purposes:
☐ Has Not Changed During Preceding 12 Months
☐ Has Changed During Preceding 12 Months (Publisher must submit explanation of change with this statement)

PS Form 3526, September 2007 (Page 1 of 3 (Instructions Page 3)) PSN 7530-01-000-9931 **PRIVACY NOTICE**: See our Privacy policy in www.usps.com

---

13. Publication Title		14. Issue Date for Circulation Data Below	
Facial Plastic Surgery Clinics of North America		May 2009	
15. Extent and Nature of Circulation		Average No. Copies Each Issue During Preceding 12 Months	No. Copies of Single Issue Published Nearest to Filing Date
a. Total Number of Copies (Net press run)		1340	1260
b. Paid Circulation (By Mail and Outside the Mail)	(1) Mailed Outside-County Paid Subscriptions Stated on PS Form 3541. (Include paid distribution above nominal rate, advertiser's proof copies, and exchange copies)	561	537
	(2) Mailed In-County Paid Subscriptions Stated on PS Form 3541 (Include paid distribution above nominal rate, advertiser's proof copies, and exchange copies)		
	(3) Paid Distribution Outside the Mails Including Sales Through Dealers and Carriers, Street Vendors, Counter Sales, and Other Paid Distribution Outside USPS®	113	105
	(4) Paid Distribution by Other Classes Mailed Through the USPS (e.g. First-Class Mail®)		
c. Total Paid Distribution (Sum of 15b (1), (2), (3), and (4))	▶	674	642
d. Free or Nominal Rate Distribution (By Mail and Outside the Mail)	(1) Free or Nominal Rate Outside-County Copies Included on PS Form 3541	100	110
	(2) Free or Nominal Rate In-County Copies Included on PS Form 3541		
	(3) Free or Nominal Rate Copies Mailed at Other Classes Through the USPS (e.g. First-Class Mail)		
	(4) Free or Nominal Rate Distribution Outside the Mail (Carriers or other means)		
e. Total Free or Nominal Rate Distribution (Sum of 15d (1), (2), (3) and (4))	▶	100	110
f. Total Distribution (Sum of 15c and 15e)	▶	774	752
g. Copies not Distributed (See instructions to publishers #4 (page #3))	▶	566	508
h. Total (Sum of 15f and g)	▶	1340	1260
i. Percent Paid (15c divided by 15f times 100)		87.08%	85.37%

16. Publication of Statement of Ownership
☐ If the publication is a general publication, publication of this statement is required. Will be printed in the November 2009 issue of this publication. ☐ Publication not required

17. Signature and Title of Editor, Publisher, Business Manager, or Owner   Date

Stephen R. Bushing   September 15, 2009
Stephen R. Bushing – Subscription Services Coordinator

I certify that all information furnished on this form is true and complete. I understand that anyone who furnishes false or misleading information on this form or who omits material or information requested on the form may be subject to criminal sanctions (including fines and imprisonment) and/or civil sanctions (including civil penalties).

PS Form 3526, September 2007 (Page 2 of 3)

Moving?

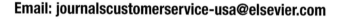

Make sure your subscription moves with you!

To notify us of your new address, find your **Clinics Account Number** (located on your mailing label above your name), and contact customer service at:

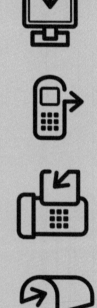

Email: journalscustomerservice-usa@elsevier.com

800-654-2452 (subscribers in the U.S. & Canada)
314-447-8871 (subscribers outside of the U.S. & Canada)

Fax number: 314-447-8029

Elsevier Health Sciences Division
Subscription Customer Service
3251 Riverport Lane
Maryland Heights, MO 63043

*To ensure uninterrupted delivery of your subscription, please notify us at least 4 weeks in advance of move.

Printed and bound by CPI Group (UK) Ltd, Croydon, CR0 4YY

03/10/2024

01040362-0011

.